THE
DISEASE
DETECTIVES

DEADLY MEDICAL MYSTERIES AND
THE PEOPLE WHO SOLVED THEM

by Gerald Astor

A PLUME BOOK

NEW AMERICAN LIBRARY

NEW YORK AND SCARBOROUGH, ONTARIO

NAL BOOKS ARE AVAILABLE AT QUANTITY DISCOUNTS WHEN USED
TO PROMOTE PRODUCTS AND SERVICES. FOR INFORMATION
PLEASE WRITE TO PREMIUM MARKETING DIVISION,
NEW AMERICAN LIBRARY, 1633 BROADWAY, NEW YORK,
NEW YORK 10019.

Library of Congress Cataloging in Publication Data

Astor, Gerald, 1926-
  The disease detectives.

  Bibliography: p.
  Includes index.
  1. Centers for Disease Control (U.S.)—History.
2. Epidemiology—Research—United States—History.
3. Epidemics—United States—History. I. Title.
RA650.5.A78 1984   616.07′1   83-26867
ISBN 0-452-25540-6

 PLUME TRADEMARK REG. U.S. PAT. OFF. AND FOREIGN COUNTRIES
REGISTERED TRADEMARK—MARCA REGISTRADA
HECHO EN HARRISONBURG, VA., U.S.A.

SIGNET, SIGNET CLASSIC, MENTOR, PLUME, MERIDIAN
and NAL BOOKS are published *in the United States* by
New American Library, 1633 Broadway, New York,
New York 10019, *in Canada* by The New American Library
of Canada Limited, 81 Mack Avenue, Scarborough,
Ontario M1L 1M8

Original hardcover edition designed by Julian Hamer

First Plume Printing, April, 1984

1 2 3 4 5 6 7 8 9

PRINTED IN THE UNITED STATES OF AMERICA

GERALD ASTOR, an editor and writer for over 25 years, has been a frequent contributor to such national magazines as *Sports Illustrated*, *Saturday Evening Post*, *Playboy*, and *Esquire*. His books include *The New York Cops* (1971), *A Question of Rape* (1974), *Hot Paper* (1975), and *Brick Agent* (1977). He currently makes his home in Scarsdale, New York.

Contents

CHAPTER

1

The CDC on the Case

GEORGE CHARPENTIER, 44, worked as a driller on offshore oil rigs along the coast of Louisiana. A strapping six-foot, 205-pound former marine who lived in the bayou country near Abbeville, Charpentier enjoyed good health until one summer morning a severe bout of diarrhea struck him. The first day Charpentier dosed himself with liberal amounts of Donnagel, an over-the-counter antidiarrheal drug. His condition did not improve. By afternoon he registered a temperature of 101°, and in spite of the August heat, chills gripped his body.

On the second day, Charpentier switched medications. But Lomotil also failed to alleviate his constant distress. On the third day, his joints aching, Charpentier tried an even more drastic substance, paregoric. "It burned terribly when I swallowed it," says Charpentier, "but it didn't help. I went to the bathroom fifteen times in a twelve-hour period. When I got on a scale I saw that I had lost 11 pounds in a single day. I went to see a doctor."

The physician was uncertain whether Charpentier was the victim of food poisoning or an intestinal virus. But the symptoms were so severe he immediately admitted Charpentier to the hospital in Abbeville.

A hospital workup found nothing exceptional in Charpentier's medical history. He recalled no stomach operations, nor was he using any medicines that might have triggered such an intensive intestinal reaction. For fifteen years he had experienced brief episodes of cramps accompanied by mild diarrhea. But a check of medical records from earlier examinations indicated that his digestive system operated well within the normal range.

Meanwhile, there was a pressing need to prevent him from going into fatal shock because he was losing fluid so rapidly. The Abbeville hospital pumped close to 13 quarts of intravenous solutions into Charpentier within four days. Doctors also prescribed strong oral antibiotic drugs, and then conducted a battery of tests. Among these were some baffling stool samples that revealed a rodlike bacterium known as serratia. It showed surprisingly little resistance to antibiotics. This is almost never the case, since serratia has always managed to stay half a jump ahead of most drugs. These bacteria have an uncanny ability to mutate, and so most serratia are a formidable challenge even to a multi-antibiotic attack.

But this particular organism, although it resembled serratia, obviously lacked that resistance. Further tests revealed that it was actually a spiral-shaped microbe, much like a comma. That unique structure belongs to a genus of organisms known as vibrios.

"We'd seen vibrios before," says Dr. Charles T. Caraway, a veterinarian and the Louisiana state epidemiologist, "and they were of no particular significance. In fact, in this instance when the report came in on a vibrio, nobody even bothered to notify me."

However, a specimen was sent to the Centers for Disease Control, the federal agency responsible for monitoring and controlling epidemics. "On a Saturday afternoon," recalls Caraway, "Roger Feldman [then chief of the Enteric Disease Branch of the CDC] called me at home and said they'd identified it as a *Vibrio cholerae* El Tor Inaba. Feldman said they were going to run it through again to make sure. But on Monday, Labor Day, he called to say there was no doubt about it. It was cholera."

Cholera. Of all the diseases known to modern humankind, cholera has been the most brutal. In periodic worldwide eruptions called pandemics, over the past 200 years cholera has slain tens of millions of people. It has ravaged the United States several times, including a visit to New Orleans in 1832 that left 5,000 dead and a repeat performance in 1849 that killed another 5,000.

The CDC immediately dispatched Dr. Paul Blake, the resident expert on cholera, to Louisiana to discover how

George Charpentier had picked up a vibrio and if there was a threat of an epidemic of the disease.

Some 7 miles from the Atlanta headquarters of the CDC lies its Center for Environmental Health in the suburb of Chamblee. The cluster of white wood-shingled one-floor buildings is a leftover from a "temporary" military hospital. It features recent additions of corrugated metal, cardboard-thin interior walls, winding passageways, and windowless cubicles. Aged government-issue desks contrast with blinking computer terminals.

Dr. Glyn Caldwell is chief of the cancer branch located in this center. On a wall near his office hangs a large map of the United States, once used for tracking sarcoma of the liver. There is a suspiciously large bunch of pins in New Jersey. A framed photograph of Great Britain's John Snow Pub, a holy place in the annals of epidemiology, graces one wall, and bulletin boards abound. Among the items on one bulletin board is a letter taken from a medical journal. It reads: "Common things occur commonly. When you hear hoofbeats, look for horses, not zebras." This is a well-loved cliché of medicine that warns young physicians against a tendency to diagnose rare diseases for ordinary symptoms. Based on this theory, the correspondent to the medical journal wrote that while visiting a science fair he heard hoofbeats and yells from an excited crowd. As an experienced hand, he naturally expected to see a runaway horse. But along came a pair of zebras with their handlers. Concluded the writer, "There is always a possibility of a zebra but one must know a zebra when he sees it."

Glyn Caldwell heard hoofbeats one morning when Dr. Jay Jacobson, a former investigator in the CDC's Epidemic Intelligence Service (EIS), called. After his work in the CDC's Special Pathogens Branch, Jacobson had accepted a fellowship in infectious diseases at the University of Utah Medical Center, and one day he was asked to look in on a 47-year-old patient in the Veterans Administration hospital.

Paul Cooper, a retired career army man, had served in both Korea and Vietnam. In spite of the outward appearance of good health, the onetime paratrooper was already a

doomed man. He had been diagnosed as having acute myelo-
blastic leukemia. He had been admitted to the VA hospital
because of a stubborn infection that developed after chemotherapy treatments.

Jacobson remembers Paul Cooper as a reasonable, articulate man. "When I looked at his medical records, I saw that
he had been exposed to radiation as a soldier participating in
tests of combat troops operating in the vicinity of above-
ground nuclear explosions in the Nevada desert during the
1950s. Cooper was quite graphic in his description of his
experiences during the tests, talking about how close to ground
zero they had marched, what it was like with the dust swirl-
ing about."

During his chat with Dr. Jacobson and subsequently in
interviews, Cooper claimed that he had been stationed in a
trench roughly 3,000 yards from ground zero, where the
bomb was located in a 700-foot high tower. The troops were
instructed to face away from the tower and cover their eyes
with their hands when the device detonated. Cooper remembered, "I could see the bones in my hands like an X-ray. The
heat was quite intense, almost unbearable for ten to twenty
seconds. We were told to turn around. We did and watched
the fireball rise into the sky." When his unit marched closer
to the site of the explosion, Cooper said, "the ground was
still cherry-hot."

Another eyewitness to the same explosion, helicopter pilot
Thomas Stedman, said, "The entire exercise area was covered with a heavy dust cloud caused by the blast. This dust
cloud extended from ground level to a height of several thousand feet." William Dillon was also a helicopter pilot at the
test, which was code-named Smokey. "The ground was like
Jell-O, but it was coming back, solidifying. We were told to
go up and land on ground zero. But we couldn't land. The
ground was like molten glass. The sand turned into glass, the
ground was so hot."

Smokey was a part of a series of A-bomb tests in Operation Plumbbob. Altogether the U.S. detonated about 200 of
these above-ground blasts in Nevada, and 300,000 U.S. soldiers were present at tests from 1948 to 1963, when a treaty
between the U.S. and the Soviet Union banned above-ground
tests.

Jay Jacobson was not privy to these details of Smokey, but he says, "The more we talked, the more curious I got about what was known of the effects of the tests on troops who were there. Cooper himself had already related his disease to the tests. I called Ed Baker, head of the then newly formed Cancer and Birth Defects Division of the CDC, a former colleague in the EIS, and asked him about it."

The sequence of events is ironic. The EIS was originally the brainchild of Dr. Alexander Langmuir, chief epidemiologist at the institution in 1949–50. The CDC lacked high-caliber epidemiologists. Langmuir wooed Congressional support by expounding on the dangers of bacteriological warfare. Creation of the EIS, reasoned Langmuir, would provide the country with a large cadre of experts whose skills could be immediately mustered in the event of a biological-warfare attack. The legislators were sufficiently impressed, and the EIS was established. Now the CDC was considering the possibility that our own weapons might have brought disease to Americans.

There was a period during the 1950s when scientists thought viruses might cause leukemia. In Niles, Illinois, eight children from a particular school developed the disease. "Clusters like that one," says Caldwell, "are the kind of oddball occurrences that offer studies of opportunity." And yet the Niles cluster turned out to be a freakish coincidence that provided no clues about leukemia.

Smokey was another opportunity for study. As Glyn Caldwell began to accumulate data, the sound of hoofbeats drummed louder and louder. But the nature of the beast, whether horse or zebra, was not yet apparent.

Yet another CDC hunting party sought to find the why of an alarming new phenomenon that showed itself first at the UCLA Medical Center in March 1981.

Donald Davis (pseudonym), 33, was examined by doctors at UCLA after having been treated by his private physician for a fever that had persisted for at least two months. The symptoms suggested a lung inflammation, a stubborn pneumonia. Davis was given a strong antibiotic, and his condition improved, temporarily. Yet a few weeks later Davis was again hospitalized. An open-lung biopsy discovered *Pneumo-*

cystis carinii pneumonia (also known as *Pneumocystis* pneumonia, *P. carinii* pneumonia, and PCP). In spite of the best in life-support systems, Davis declined rapidly and died.

PCP is an uncommon disease, but oddly enough Davis was the second victim at UCLA that spring. A 30-year-old man, Howard Andrews (pseudonym), with a four-month history of fever and malaise, had been treated at UCLA for PCP after bronchial brushings revealed traces of the malady. In Davis's case, the doctors decided to use a drug called pentamadine. "This is a highly toxic preparation," remarks Dr. James Curran of the CDC, who was shortly to become head of the task force assigned to the matter. "In 100 percent of the times it is used there are side effects. It is rarely employed as a result and happens to be one of the few items exclusively obtained through the CDC." The requisition for pentamadine thus informed the CDC of a case of PCP.

About the same time, Dr. Wayne Shandera, an EIS officer posted in Los Angeles, was chatting with an allergist who taught at UCLA. The professor remarked on the strange coincidence of two cases of PCP. He suggested that Shandera see about publicizing the matter through the medium of a CDC weekly report, the *Morbidity and Mortality Weekly Report (MMWR)*. Shandera routinely checked other hospitals for similar manifestations. To the EIS officer's astonishment, he discovered that within a few months, three other men had been diagnosed as suffering from PCP, and one had died. All five patients, men under age 40, were active homosexuals, although they did not know one another, nor did they have common contacts or sexual partners with a similar disease.

Shortly after Shandera compiled this information, the 37-year-old Curran traveled from Atlanta to San Diego for a seminar on VD control. During the meeting, brief mention was made of the peculiar circumstances of the five PCP cases. "After one session," recalls Curran, "some doctors from San Francisco's Bay Area Gay Physicians group approached me. They said PCP was not the only new medical problem for gays. They told me they had seen recently several instances of a rare tumor, Kaposi's sarcoma. I'd never seen a case, never heard of it before."

Indeed, if one checks the index of a standard physician's desk reference book, like the *Merck Manual*, he won't find a listing for Kaposi's sarcoma. It is a form of skin cancer originally associated with Eastern Europeans, particularly Jews from that area. Kaposi himself was originally named Cohen. He switched to a less ethnic surname in order to overcome the rampant anti-Semitism of Austria-Hungary in the 1870s and obtain the post of professor of dermatology in Vienna.

"The literature on Kaposi's," explains Curran, "shows that in the previous records on the disease, out of 100 U.S. cases, 85 percent of the patients were over 65 and at most six deaths in a hundred cases could be attributed to Kaposi's. But these doctors from San Francisco were talking in terms of much younger men and a much higher rate of fatalities.

"You see Kaposi's in people who've been immuno-suppressed, renal-transplant patients who've taken drugs to prevent rejection of the new kidney as alien tissue, or in cancer patients whose immune system has been knocked out by chemotherapy. Cancer registries show that among immuno-suppressed patients, KS is 3 percent of the cancers. It is 2 to 4 percent in transplant patients and only .02 percent of the cancers that appear in otherwise healthy people." The figures tumble from Curran's lips quickly; for a man who had never heard of the disease a few weeks earlier, he had obviously done considerable studying.

"There is one exception, at least until now, in parts of Africa, where Kaposi's sarcoma is fairly common in younger guys and there are a high number of deaths from the disease.

"Kaposi's is not something that's quickly noticed. A guy will be feeling ill for six or eight months with no particular complaint. The visible sign is a purplish lesion, a slightly raised discoloration something like a bruise. It may be smaller than a penny, show anywhere on the body. Ordinarily it's the kind of thing that might be seen in a dermatologist's office. It's frequently misdiagnosed, and it isn't something that sends a person to a hospital. People don't usually die from Kaposi's."

P. carinii pneumonia has one thing in common with KS. It too is ordinarily associated with an underlying condition that has somehow destroyed the individual's immune system. "Historically," says Curran, "PCP almost always was connected with an underlying condition that lowered resistance. Of 194 previous cases we looked at, this was true in 193 of them."

In view of these reports, the CDC immediately contacted health-monitoring agencies, hospitals, and specialists who might have come across either PCP or KS to determine whether some strange new disease problem afflicted gays or if the phenomenon was just another inexplicable oddity like the Niles, Illinois, cluster of leukemia fruitlessly investigated by Glyn Caldwell.

New York sources reported that physicians there had indeed been puzzled by the appearance of a number of cases of both diseases and that the victims were youthful gay males.

"We flew to New York right away to see people at Sloan Kettering [a hospital specializing in cancer] and New York University Hospital, where many of the men had been treated," says Curran. "We visited some of the patients. It was very difficult talking to a dying gay. One man, little, shriveled, and dying, had been married and then was divorced about fifteen years ago. He had made a deathbed request that his sons, now well established in professions, come to see him. They refused. Some of the patients were men who had successfully hidden their gay life from their wives, parents, and other relatives, and now in their sickness it was revealed. There was a tremendous amount of emotional pain and in some instances guilt, a sense that their way of life had caused the disease."

One victim presented subsequently was a kind of classic illustration of the condition. Call him Robert Watson; he was originally from Philadelphia, in his mid-30s, gay, and before his illness quite obese, weighing close to 290 pounds. He had first become ill in November 1980 when he developed a shortness of breath, although there was no evidence of any heart disease or respiratory sickness. Admitted to a hospital, he lost 50 or 60 pounds with no change in his symptoms. Discharged from the hospital, he continued to lose weight, and by March 1981 he was down to 195 pounds. He returned to the hospital for further examination and on this occasion he was diagnosed as having *P. carinii* pneumonia. Treatment seemed to alleviate the condition, and he left the hospital, only to check in two months later with severe diarrhea. He weighed in at 170, and lab tests revealed an infection with several organisms. In spite of treatment, the symptoms continued, and the patient decided to move to Florida. He continued to be sick, and over this period of time there were some changes in his personality. Doctors decided that his trouble was a mental illness. "This is an unfortunate way of some physicians," says Curran. "The chronically ill, unexplainable disease is the bane of physicians. The feeling is, 'If I can't cure him, he must be crazy.'"

Made aware of the CDC's interest in gay men with PCP, Watson moved to Atlanta and checked into Emory University Hospital, just up the road from the CDC. He now weighed 139 pounds, less than half of his original level. "He had what looked like a yeast infection," says Curran, who examined him, "and it called for some dramatic systemic treatment," meaning very strong drugs. "When we looked in his mouth we discovered two small purple lesions on the hard palate; a biopsy showed he had Kaposi's sarcoma. He was going downhill like a starving man. For some inexplicable reason his immune system had been suppressed and the condition appeared irreversible. Any drugs given to deal with his infection could only suppress his resistance to disease even further."

Curran no longer had any doubts that there was a real problem, that he was dealing with a genuine epidemic. The critical question was why it targeted a particular group of people.

John and Eleanor Kiley had begun a vacation drive through the southeastern states with an ultimate destination of St. Augustine, Florida, and Disney World. Home was Fort Washington, Pennsylvania, where the 57-year-old, gray-haired Kiley worked as a drill-press operator, followed the fortunes of baseball's Phillies, and devoted much of his spare time to the local post of the American Legion. During World War II, John Kiley had served as a medic. He was a man of plain tastes, fond of meat and potatoes, and in the words of his wife had grown "a little potbelly from drinking beer."

Eleanor Kiley had been somewhat reluctant to start their trip. Her husband was definitely off his feed and had confessed that he felt very tired. Apparently, the state convention of Legionnaires which Kiley had just attended in Philadelphia had fatigued him. His health was only fair. Three years before he had suffered a mild heart attack, and twenty-five years before he had rammed his car into a tree. At that time a priest had given him the last rites. But although his leg was broken in several places, Kiley had survived. However, the accident left him with a residue, a stiff-legged walk and pain whenever he spent much time on his feet.

In Philadelphia, Kiley's leg and a mild malaise bothered him enough so that he passed up a final evening of partying with his Legionnaire roommates staying at the Bellevue Stratford Hotel. He remained in the room for a night, eating a few crackers and watching television.

When Kiley arrived home from the convention, he and his wife ate dinner at their daughter's house, next door. Kiley did not finish his plate of macaroni and cheese. He announced, "I'm tired," and walked home to sleep. He still lacked his usual zest the following day but reported to his wife that he had neither a sore throat nor a stomachache.

On Monday night, the eve of their departure for the South, Eleanor Kiley prepared a favorite meal of her husband's: pork chops, mashed potatoes, salad, and iced tea. He poked about the food, left some on his plate. When his wife suggested they delay their trip, he insisted they leave on schedule. A rush visit to the dry cleaner retrieved a leisure suit that had seen service at the American Legion convention, and it was included in the final packing.

On Tuesday, with Eleanor Kiley behind the wheel, they traveled all the way to Rocky Mount, North Carolina. On Wednesday morning they paused for breakfast. John Kiley downed three half-pint containers of milk, which surprised his wife. He was ordinarily not a milk drinker.

By lunchtime they had covered another 158 miles and halted at a Howard Johnson restaurant in Dillon, South Carolina. After looking over the menu with a notable absence of enthusiasm, Kiley ordered only a dish of apple sauce. The waitress replied that item was not available. Kiley settled for a portion of mashed potatoes. He had barely swallowed a mouthful before he gagged. Thoroughly alarmed, Eleanor Kiley decided they would go no farther without seeing a doctor. Unable to locate one immediately, Mrs. Kiley drove her husband to the emergency room of St. Eugene's Community Hospital.

The patient presenting himself at the emergency room appeared to Dr. J. Budding, the doctor on duty, to be run-down, possibly on the verge of pneumonia, and as a side note, "a man who looked like he enjoyed a drink." The niceties of hospital procedure required that Kiley be seen by a physician in private practice before he could be admitted to St. Eugene's. Budding telephoned Dr. Blake Berry, a 30-year-old former Green Beret having lunch at his home.

When Berry met Kiley, the Pennsylvanian asked only for an antibiotic that would enable him and his wife to continue their journey. But after Berry examined Kiley it was agreed that for safety's sake it would be wise to hospitalize the traveler and treat him as a pneumonia patient. Eleanor Kiley moved into a local hotel while her husband took up residence at St. Eugene's and began to receive an antibiotic.

On Thursday, Kiley, who had become unable to swallow in the interim, ate some soft foods and appeared alert. But his condition was not satisfactory to Blake Berry. "I expected an improvement and a decrease in fever." Instead, Kiley's temperature stood at 102° and his chest had become congested. He started to cough.

Later that same day, Kiley's health deteriorated considerably. "He raved," said Mrs. Kiley. "He said we shouldn't forget a wedding on Saturday. We were on vacation for two weeks. There was no wedding."

Berry ordered extensive lab tests on the patient's blood, urine, and sputum. They offered no clue to the cause of his sickness. The physician prescribed a higher dose of antibiotics. "I expected a clinical response by Friday afternoon," said Berry. Instead, Kiley's fever rose to 103.5°. He had difficulty breathing. Sometimes he was lucid; other periods he spoke nonsense.

"I had never lost a patient to pneumonia," recalls Berry. "I would lie awake at night trying to figure out why he didn't respond."

Nothing seemed to work, not the antibiotics and not the oxygen administered. Berry had the unhappy task of informing Eleanor Kiley of the danger to her husband's life. She tried to assume an optimistic stance, saying, "This man has had a tough life. He has pneumonia but he's going to fight it off." She was, however, not reassured during a visit to him on Saturday. "His hands were ice-cold. His face had a purplish color," a sign of insufficient oxygenated blood.

On Sunday the Kileys' daughter and son-in-law arrived in Dillon. "He may have known we were all there," says his wife. "He opened his eyes slightly." But although an X-ray indicated a slight improvement in his chest congestion, John Kiley died at 11:55 p.m.

"Why I lost him I don't know," said Berry at the time. "For all I know, he had pneumonia."

On Monday morning, August 2, the day after John Kiley succumbed to what appeared to be an intractable case of pneumonia, Dr. Robert Sharrar, the bearded, bespectacled chief of the Communicable Diseases Control Section of the Philadelphia Health Department, walked to his office in the downtown area of the city. Following his usual route, Sharrar's path took him down Broad Street past the Bellevue Stratford Hotel, a 70-year-old fixture of the city and the site of the recently concluded American Legion convention. In his mid-30s, Sharrar was oblivious to the bay-windowed seventeen-story hotel, which was to become so much a focus of his life in weeks to come. The epidemiologist was preoccupied with the coming birth of his first child.

Sharrar was hardly at his desk, however, when he received a telephone call from Dr. William Parkin, a veterinarian, doctor of public health, and then acting epidemiologist for the state. Parkin, calling from his post in the state capital, Harrisburg, informed Sharrar, "We've had eleven deaths from pneumonia and every case attended the American Legion convention last week in Philadelphia."

Sharrar still remembers his feeling of horror. For months there had been predictions of a swine flu epidemic; a swine flu outbreak in 1918 had killed 20 million around the world, 500,000 in the United States. He said despairingly, "If it's swine flu, then we're finished. We didn't have time to get everyone immunized. The whole country's going to get it."

Pennsylvania operates a well-funded, well-trained public health organization. But authorities like Sharrar and Parkin recognized that they lacked the resources to combat a severe epidemic. The Pennsylvania health officials, like their counterparts who faced cholera, possible radiation sickness, and the gay men's epidemic, turned to the CDC.

At the time Legionnaires' disease erupted in Philadelphia, the CDC table of organization in Atlanta actually listed a single center surrounded by satellite bureaus covering a number of public health services. In 1980 the institution was restructured into six operational units, five of which bear the designation "center."

The Center for Infectious Diseases serves as the umbrella for more than a dozen sections concerned with different elements of communicable illnesses. Its experts tracked a mysterious malady that slew Laotian refugees in their sleep. Its specialists in gastrointestinal ailments rush to cruise ships buffeted by waves of food poisoning. The same unit maintains a constant watch for that scourge from the Far East, cholera. Viral-disease scientists deal with that common specimen, measles, and also monitor incredibly lethal hemorrhagic fevers, agents so deadly that they require a special facility known as the Maximum Containment Laboratory. There the staff labors in a science-fiction atmosphere to avoid either falling victim themselves or permitting the deadly specimens to escape.

This center also features a Special Pathogens Branch, a kind of catchall for diseases of unknown origins. It went on the case when women suddenly became vulnerable to a frightening condition known as toxic shock. Offshoots of this branch patrol U.S. territory where a relic from 600 years ago, the black death—bubonic plague—lurks and where other insect-borne enemies of human health thrive.

The Center for Prevention Services oversees control of tuberculosis, and operates quarantine stations that play a prominent role in restriction of imported diseases. It is also responsible for national immunization programs. On the doorstep of this center was laid the great swine-flu fiasco. Prevention Services includes the battle against gonorrhea and syphilis, both increasingly resistant to antibiotics. The effort has been complicated by the wildfire spread of herpes, a sexually transmitted viral infection. This unit also addressed itself to the mysterious appearance of two deadly nonvenereal diseases among gay men.

The Center for Health Promotion and Education provides surveillance and investigation into abortion phenomena, like a recent, startling cluster of spontaneous miscarriages among department-store employees.

The Center for Environmental Health focuses on environmentally related diseases and chronic ailments such as cancer. Medical detectives from this center study soldiers who participated in the Nevada atomic-bomb tests, babies in Tennessee with a rare illness, and the dumping of asbestos tailings at a housing site in Arizona.

A fifth unit, the Center for Professional Development and Training, provides in-house programs for the elevation of skills and knowledge. The last of the operational units is the National Institute for Occupational Safety and Health (NIOSH), devoted to safety and health standards in job situations. NIOSH's recommendations are implemented by the Occupational Safety and Health Agency (OSHA).

An Epidemiology Program Office recruits and assigns new talent for the CDC, young men and women who are posted for two-year stints at health units across the country. EIS officers are actually on a par with officers in the armed forces. Service in the EIS is accepted in lieu of military obligations. At any given time the EIS numbers about a hundred health professionals, mainly doctors but with a smattering of Ph.Ds, nurses, and scientists.

The Epidemiology Program Office also collects national health statistics and publishes information on investigations in its *Morbidity and Mortality Weekly Report (MMWR)*.

Through an International Health Program Office, the CDC assigns specialists to work abroad on such frightening agents as Africa's hemorrhagic viruses.

Overall, the CDC employs close to 4,000 people—doctors, microbiologists, toxologists, veterinarians, technicians, and support staff. The CDC operates fifteen laboratories with more than 250,000 of the bacterial, viral, and rickettsial enemies of human well-being on file. Some labs demand special credentials for admission. Entry to the Maximum Containment Lab requires vaccination against a number of exotic diseases.

At the Atlanta headquarters are a batch of administrators and a director, currently Dr. William Foege, himself a leader in the worldwide effort that extinguished smallpox.

About half of the CDC staff are stationed in Atlanta, most of them working in a complex of buildings near Emory University in the Druid Hills section of the city. Headquarters is a nondescript off-white brick edifice, seven stories high. A bust of Hygeia, the Greek goddess of health, stands out in front.

Each CDC hunt begins with a different focus. For example, in the matter of George Charpentier, the puzzle was how. In the matter of the famous investigation of Legionnaires' disease, the question was what—what was actually causing the disease? The gay men's disease asked: Why? And Glyn Caldwell's conundrum for those at nuclear tests was: Whether?

CHAPTER

2

"One of the Most Dangerous Things in the World"

"WHATEVER IT IS, it is one of the most dangerous things in the world." These were the words of Dr. Jay Satz, chief virologist of Pennsylvania, as Legionnaires' disease casualties mounted. Ordinarily Philadelphia would see twenty to thirty pneumonia deaths a week from its entire population of a million. But at the time the CDC was called, the eleven pneumonia deaths among a group of 5,000 Legionnaires were an extraordinarily high attack rate.

Robert Sharrar, who had done a two-year stint in the EIS before taking his post in Philadelphia, recalls, "That afternoon [following the notification from Parkin], there were two more deaths, several more cases, and a co-worker of mine was displaying the same symptoms. He hadn't even been at the convention but he walked past the Bellevue Stratford," as indeed had Sharrar that morning.

The disease also ravaged the stately Bellevue Stratford Hotel at the city's center. The hotel, with its marble-walled lobby, gold-leafed columns, and baroque mirrors, no longer reverberated with the bustling camaraderie of conventioneers, business travelers, and tourists. Instead it took on the hushed quiet of a hospital. Most of the 750 rooms emptied out as reservations went unfilled; thirty gatherings scheduled for the next few months were canceled. Bellevue Stratford bellhops reported that women refused to date them because of their association with the plague spot. President Gerald Ford, in an effort to allay anxiety, refused to skip his appearance at the Eucharistic Congress in Philadelphia. But business and social life in the city suffered. Commuters brown-bagged it to their offices in Philadelphia rather than risk eating at any restaurant, particularly those in the Bellevue Stratford. Fans stayed away from games of the baseball Phillies.

The fear was not confined to Philadelphia. "Nobody will come to our house. They're all scared to death," said Emma Dixon of Jeanette, Pennsylvania, whose husband was one of the lucky Legionnaires who managed to recover from the disease. In Williamstown, a physician's secretary attended a Little League game. Other mothers quickly moved away from her seat; they knew her boss was treating victims of the savage disease. New York City reported that its preventable-disease bureau was swamped with calls from people worried about relatives and friends from Pennsylvania and the chances of the scourge traveling to New York.

Hospitals and funeral parlors filled up. Sam Morris, 48, a Korean War vet, had stayed at the Bellevue Stratford, but like John Kiley, feeling ill, passed up the final festivities. Feeling terrible after he drove home to Lime Ridge, Pennsylvania, Morris telephoned Dr. Ernest Campbell. The physician took no chances after examining Morris. He had him admitted to the Bloomsburg Hospital. When his patient casually remarked that two buddies who had attended the convention with him were also in the hospital, Campbell checked on them. His suspicions were aroused by the similarity of the symptoms of all three men. Campbell alerted the local office of the state health department, making him probably the first to discover the outbreak of the epidemic. But one of Morris's companions was already beyond help, dying of "acute lung failure."

Meanwhile, 50 miles away in Williamsport, there were six patients in the hospital, all from the American Legion meeting and all with the same sinister symptoms. The information was relayed to state health authorities. By Monday it was clear that an epidemic had erupted, and Robert Sharrar received the telephone call from Dr. William Parkin.

Dr. David Fraser, an affable, tall, slender man in his mid-30s and a former EIS officer himself, had been named to direct the CDC's task force. His investigators from the CDC (more than thirty were sent eventually) and local authorities set up a "war room" in Harrisburg to pool and analyze data. "There were actually two rooms," says Fraser. "One was for the epidemiologists and the other was staffed by public-health personnel, secretaries, Philadelphia cops, and EIS officers who answered all of the calls from those who were concerned about the disease." On the wall of the room with the epidemiologists was a large map of the state with yellow pins to chart cases, red ones to denote death. By the end of the first full day of operations, the task force had run out of yellow markers as more than seventy cases were confirmed. There were already eighteen red pins to remind the team of the enemy's deadly nature.

The experts quickly agreed upon a rough case definition. It consisted of a cough and fever of 102° F. or higher, or any fever and chest X-ray evidence of pneumonia. The victims also had to have had some association with the American Legion convention—either actual attendance or coming within one block of headquarters, the ill-fated Bellevue Stratford.

During the following three days, EIS officers fanned out from Pittsburgh, Harrisburg, and Philadelphia to interview and examine known cases. The investigators averaged 450 miles of driving as they sought out patients in half a dozen hospitals. Dr. Stephen Thacker of the EIS, wearing a yellow mask, gown, and gloves, stood at the bedside of the 43-year-old Sydney Easter in Harrisburg General Hospital. Having reviewed Easter's chart, Thacker asked if the sick Legionnaire had attended the Keystone "Go Better Breakfast" at the Bellevue Stratford. Had he gone to the dinner at the Benjamin Franklin Hotel, had he drunk from containers in the hotel ballrooms, and had he had any recent contact with pigs? Swine flue dominated the early list of suspects.

When Dr. David Sencer, then director of the CDC, first met with the investigators being dispatched from Atlanta, he had mentioned the possibility of swine flu but was careful to warn against any premature conclusions. The CDC is responsible for tracking recurrent assaults by flu viruses and initiating immunization programs. Toward the end of 1975 and early in 1976, several individuals in New Jersey, including a soldier at Fort Dix who died, contracted a different form of flu. From their blood serum (the amber-colored fluid that remains in blood after clotting elements are removed), antibodies that seemed identical to those harbored by people who had survived the great 1918 swine flu pandemic were recovered. That outbreak had killed as many as 500,000 Americans, 20 million people around the world. Top officials at the CDC, including Sencer, had been convinced that the next year would see swine flu in the U.S. The CDC had asked for a government-sponsored swine flu immunization effort.

The swine flu theory received a boost with the report that three victims had lived only 10 miles from the home of the GI who had died of what was tentatively diagnosed as that form of the disease. Like Sharrar, David Fraser was most apprehensive that they were up against swine flu. To manufacture and distribute vaccine and reach the public would take months. Even then, ten to fourteen days must elapse before the vaccine could provide adequate protection. By then the toll could be incalculable.

The possibility of swine flu, however, collapsed by August 10. The EIS officers who canvassed the patients and their survivors realized that Legionnaires' disease appeared self-limiting. "The number of new cases was dramatically down," says Sharrar. "Whatever it was did not involve any secondary cases. People in the hospital and the family were not developing the disease. It wasn't being passed from person to person [an essential characteristic of flu]. I was immensely relieved when the reports on influenza virus cultures came back negative."

Sharrar was typical of the professionals who found themselves in the front lines of the fight against Legionnaires' disease. As a medical student he had obtained a fellowship to West Pakistan, where he discovered community medicine through the work at the mission hospital. Like many of his contemporaries he was attracted to the CDC as an alternative to military service. "It was in 1965, and everyone was getting drafted after med school," says Sharrar, "and sent to Vietnam. I was told I could substitute time in the U.S. Public Health Service for medical duty and of the opportunities in the EIS."

There was another attraction to the EIS. Some members admit that as kids they had ambitions for the life of a private eye or a policeman; the EIS officers have often been labeled "disease detectives," and Sharrar once said, "If I weren't permitted to work in medicine, I'd like to be an investigative reporter."

Sharrer fell under the spell of Dr. Alexander Langmuir,

who served as chief epidemiologist of the CDC until his retirement in 1970. From Langmuir, Sharrar learned, "All of your education you've been taught to think of the individual patient. Now you must learn to think of the whole population as your patient."

That indeed was what Sharrar, Fraser, and the other investigators now attempted—to identify what menaced the entire population. For by August 10, the yellow pins denoting cases of the disease added up to 180. The deaths, marked in red, totaled twenty-nine.

Pathology reports were grim. The autopsy report of one of the dead noted that his lungs looked like steel wool. Frustrated local physicians talked like Blake Berry when he lost John Kiley. After 66-year-old cabdriver Harold Davis died, a physician confessed, "We're backed against the wall in this situation. No one knows what Davis had and no one knew how to treat him."

Dr. Leonard Bachman, the Pennsylvania state secretary of health, after looking over the statistics, considered asking for the imposition of martial law and a quarantine. "We thought we might be faced with an unprecedented condition in modern medicine, one for which we had no really effective antibiotics, drugs, or therapy."

"We were all extremely puzzled," Dr. David Heymann of the EIS says. "I went to central Pennsylvania, Reading, Allentown. Most of the patients I saw there were in desperate shape, on life-support systems. They were unable to talk to me. All of them were kept in extreme isolation; if any other person was in a bed in the room, he had the same disease."

Steve Thacker was disappointed with the results of his interviews. "Nothing seemed to add up. Some people slept near open windows, others did not. Some went out in crowds, others seem to have spent the convention in their hotel rooms. Even in the hospitals, the attitudes differed. In some they took every possible precaution with patients, placing them in isolation, all personnel capped and gowned. At another hospital the only special treatment was to wear gloves."

Walter Orenstein, a CDC measles specialist drafted for the campaign against the Philadelphia epidemic, says, "The major question we debated in the beginning was whether we were dealing with a confined outbreak, just Legionnaires around the Bellevue Stratford, or was it something citywide or even larger."

Adding to the puzzlement were some curious details. While most of the victims were Legionnaires who had attended the festivities at the Bellevue Stratford, there were thirty-eight cases who had never entered the hotel. Their closest association had been to walk within a block of the place. And then there was the oddity that not a single employee of the hotel had come down with the disease.

In all the confusion it was inevitable that rumors and false leads would abound. High anxiety gripped the public when it was reported that a busload of people who had been at the convention on the road to Georgia and that several riders had become ill. The story was unfounded.

An executive of the American Legion's rival organization, the Veterans of Foreign Wars, charged that a left-wing conspiracy had been responsible for the epidemic. He received space in the newspapers, but law-enforcement authorities dismissed the accusation. There was talk of a mystery man who might have dumped a noxious substance into the local water supply. Composite drawings of the phantom were distributed, but he was only a creature of vivid imaginations.

One woman who had been in residence at the Bellevue Stratford swore that she heard the constant chirping of parakeets. The information implied psittacosis, a disease with symptoms akin to those of the sick Legionnaires. No parakeets or other birds could be located. A terrified youth confessed that during the magicians' convention that had preceded the Legionnaires' convention at the Bellevue Stratford, he had as a prank tossed some magician's smoke powder into a hotel vent. Someone mentioned a woman who frequented the vicinity of the Bellevue Stratford feeding pigeons. The "pigeon lady," as she was inevitably dubbed, was tracked down, examined as a possible carrier of some illness, and declared innocent.

There were also a number of more scientifically based possibilities. The blood of one patient showed a substantial increase in typhoid fever antibodies. But no physicians reported typhoid's standard rose-colored spots on the chest and stomach. Nor could the distinctive typhoid bacillus be seen in the samples of tissue drawn from victims. The spike in typhoid antibodies occurred because most of the sick were military veterans who had routinely been inoculated against that disease while in service. Elevated fever triggered the response.

The investigators sifted through an encyclopedia of candidates: chlamydia, a fungal infection; histoplasmosis, an infection stemming from the inhalation of dust containing spores of a fungus; blastomycosis, a disease from a yeastlike fungus that affects skin, lungs, and the body as a whole; the parainfluenza viruses, which generally are restricted to children and usually have mild consequences; adenoviruses, a series of fevers but of a mild variety; herpes virus; mumps; measles; salmonella, a common intestinal infection; whooping cough; tularemia or rabbit fever; bubonic plague, the famed black death of medieval Europe; Marburg and Lassa fevers, hemorrhagic diseases indigenous to Africa (David Fraser had worked on a Lassa fever control project); and others.

From the living victims of the disease, the scientists took samples of blood, urine, feces, spinal fluid, and sputum. Bacteriologists placed these in nutrient broths and waited for the bacteria to grow. Virologists squinted at living cells under microscopes, hoping to detect the lethal invader. Tissues from lungs, liver, spleen, and other organs were sliced from the dead. Some specimens went under immediate scrutiny; others were carefully preserved for future study. There was a steady flow of material to the CDC labs in Atlanta, where experts like Dr. Charles Shepherd and Dr. Joseph McDade, who specialized in organisms known as rickettsia, searched for the agent responsible for the disease. But the identity of the organism remained hidden.

CDC investigators distributed two-page questionnaires to more than 1,000 American Legion posts in Pennsylvania. Some 3,683 men cooperated, an astonishingly high response. Data on who ate, drank, and breathed what and where was collected.

The media, whose first stories had been so helpful in locating victims like John Kiley, became impatient with the pace of the investigation—the process of isolation and culture of organisms from the tissues of victims may take weeks. "The press was all over the place," says Walter Orenstein. "It was difficult to discuss anything without them being involved. We were accused of withholding information when the fact was we didn't know anything to tell them."

The media could hardly be blamed for their frustration. Contradictory statements were the rule of the day. State Secretary of Health Bachman publicly attributed the epidemic to a virus rather than a bacterium on the grounds that the latter usually are easily detectable in the labs of hospitals. State Chief Virologist Jay Satz, however, declared it was 99 percent certain that the cause was not a virus.

With both viral and bacterial infections seemingly eliminated from contention, the only other possibility was a toxic substance, a poison that somehow had found its way into the food, beverages, or air consumed by the Legionnaires. A toxin explained the absence of person-to-person contagion and the strong association with a single hotel and area of the city.

Says Sharrar, "I first thought it must be airborne, but it's hard to imagine a toxin you could inhale without being aware of the odor. And if something was in the air, why didn't the staff at the Bellevue Stratford get ill? And if it were airborne, then we would probably have seen a very high attack rate."

Experts went over the Bellevue Stratford in microscopic detail, examining air conditioners, elevators, carpets, furnishings, wallpaper, and ventilating systems. Philadelphia inspectors discovered nineteen violations of the plumbing code. "It was one more red herring," says Fraser. "These had no discernible connection with the disease."

The investigators looked at the containers of water in the Grand Ballroom, but found nothing untoward. There were questions about the Bloody Marys mixed in pitchers made with a cadmium surface and the cadmium-coated ice trays. Cadmium poisoning has flu-like symptoms. However, that toxin acts far more swiftly than the sickness that had struck the Legionnaires.

Dr. F. William Sunderman, Jr., headed a team at the University of Connecticut which discovered an elevated level of nickel carbonyl in the tissues of some of the dead. Hopes that the mystery was solved collapsed quickly when further study showed that knives and utensils employed for the autopsies contained nickel carbonyl. To avoid future contamination,

Eastern Airlines supplied plastic equipment ordinarily used for serving meals on planes.

"Someone thought it might be paraquat, the stuff used on marijuana," recalls Orenstein. Paraquat, a weed killer, had been sprayed recently on weedy vegetation near the hotel. "We couldn't find any traces of paraquat," says Orenstein, "nor any reason to believe the victims might have come into contact with it."

There were suggestions that untraceable poisons had been stolen from the bacteriological-weapons labs at Fort Detrick, Maryland. "I met with people from Fort Detrick and experts on chemical warfare from Edgewood Arsenal," says Fraser. "I asked them if they were aware of any toxin that might cause an epidemic like this. They said none they knew of. All of our book reading about chemical warfare indicated that our epidemic did not match the known effects of any toxin."

About this time, criticisms of the CDC rose several decibels. The CDC was accused of having wrongly skewed the investigation because of a bias in favor of a viral cause, swine flu. As a consequence, vital information pinpointing a bacterium or a toxin was lost.

Congressman John Murphy of New York, later convicted as an ABSCAM bribe, announced, "It appears to be the consensus of opinion that the failure to save, take, and keep free from contamination the tissues of the victims of the epidemic is clearly the reason that the ultimate resolution of the Legionnaires' disease may never be found."

In truth, evidence on toxicity was restricted because many of the first victims had already been buried before anyone realized that more was involved than a routine but stubborn attack of pneumonia. Critical samples of blood, urine, and tissue were no longer obtainable from these people. Once laid to rest, the body tends to break down rapidly and shed alien substances. And in some instances, the grieving survivors refused to permit a complete postmortem examination.

Newspaper articles, including one written by a former EIS officer, chided the investigators for missing clues. "There were some low blows," remarks Orenstein. "We supposedly botched things by not getting on to toxins quickly enough. There was an assumption that we didn't know enough about toxins and if we had been competent in that field we could have found the cause."

"I didn't really feel the heat until I testified at the Congressional hearings in Philadelphia," says Fraser, speaking of the forum at which Rep. Murphy aired his beliefs. "Congressman Murphy and the others were nasty and accusatory mainly about the question of obtaining specimens for toxin testing. But the premium for everyone was on the living and making certain that the epidemic was controlled. In retrospect we didn't do a good job in terms of screening for a toxin. We should have collected more urine specimens."

None of the toxin possibilities proved out, however, and Legionnaires' disease moved to the back pages of newspapers and disappeared from the media entirely.

There was, however, one last victim. The Bellevue Stratford, with electric wiring designed by Thomas Edison himself, had been gasping for its life since the epidemic began. In spite of its gracious amenities, the hotel was now regarded as a pesthole. Nevertheless, the CDC team in Philadelphia had stayed there. "It was convenient," says David Heymann. "We were right at hand to bleed employees for tests." That was hardly the kind of endorsement calculated to improve business. By October, the occupancy rate had fallen from an average of 80 percent to a paltry 3 percent with losses of $10,000 a day.

Local movers and shakers sought to resuscitate the institution with a $50-a-plate get-well party in the main ballroom. The American Medical Association still planned to hold its convention at the hotel in December, the American Lung Association had scheduled a one-day conference on Legionnaires' disease at the Bellevue Stratford, and the Society of the Source, a parapsychology group, met there to declare the Bellevue Stratford not responsible for the epidemic, but nevertheless the hotel died in November. Subsequently, after $20 million was spent in refurbishing, the place was reborn as the Fairmount.

Meanwhile, the task force on Legionnaires' disease was dispersed. CDC director David Sencer responded to questions, "What we know is mostly what we don't know." And Alexander Langmuir, founder of the EIS, declared the affair "the greatest epidemiological puzzle of the century."

The only man still totally consumed by the investigation was David Fraser. He had discovered epidemiology in his second year at Harvard Medical School with a summer job investigating the background of Parkinsonism. One of Fraser's teachers at Harvard was himself an EIS alumnus, and it took little urging to persuade Fraser to apply for an appointment following a stint as an intern and resident, ironically at a Philadelphia hospital.

Thinking back to the winter of 1976–77, Fraser remarks, "I'd despaired that we'd solve it. The higher-ups at the CDC are very good at not applying pressure, but I felt it from time to time in people's looks, people who knew I was on the project. Mostly, my professional ego suffered terribly during these months." Understandably, many of the investigators, having gone down so many blind alleys and stumped for lack of leads, were losing their enthusiasm and energy for continued pursuit. Fraser saw part of his job as "pestering people" to keep the pace up. There had been a few unexplained substances seen in the sera from some of the victims, and Fraser placed some slim hopes upon researchers in clinical chemistry.

In December 1976, David Fraser, dressed in work boots and a tieless dress shirt, distributed copies of a proposed seventy-page report on the investigation to date. One copy went to the Leprosy and Rickettsial Disease Laboratory, directed by a veteran of the CDC, Dr. Charles Shepherd, and a newcomer, Dr. Joseph McDade. "I had worked with Shep on a leprosy matter," says Fraser," and I thought there was an outside chance that some new rickettsial agent was involved."

Charles Shepherd was 63 that December, but could easily have passed for twenty years younger. Wiry, with the leathery taut skin of a dedicated runner, Shepherd is a native of Nebraska. "My father was a doctor," says Shepherd, "and when I entered Stanford as an undergraduate, I had no thought of medicine. But he talked me into taking a premed course that first year. The Depression was on and I realized that while jobs were going to be hard to get, a doctor could always find work, so I stuck with medicine." Even when Shepherd finished his studies he was concerned enough about the economic state of the country to opt for the security of a government post in the Public Health Service. "There was a war coming on," recalls Shepherd, "and I spent that first year working on VD. But after Pearl Harbor there was a realization that the military would be engaged in places where rickettsial diseases were most common. I was assigned to work on the problem."

Rickettsial organisms fall somewhere between bacteria and viruses. Like bacteria, rickettsiae can survive and multiply outside of a living cell. Viruses, on the other hand, must be harbored by a viable cell before they can grow. Rickettsiae are far smaller than bacteria and have their own peculiar configurations. They are visible through specific slide-staining and microscopic-viewing techniques. The rickettsia family is responsible for typhus, Rocky Mountain spotted fever, and Q fever. The class of organism was discovered early in this century by Howard Ricketts, an American pathologist. While studying typhus in Mexico City in 1911, Ricketts caught the disease and died.

Shepherd's work in rickettsiae is world-renowned. In 1975, he convinced his superiors that the CDC required the services of another full-time rickettsiologist. He chose Joe McDade. The 37-year-old McDade had earned a Ph.D. from the University of Delaware and had spent two years stationed at Fort Detrick, where he studied rickettsiae. On his return to civilian life he had specialized in rickettsiae for various organizations in Cairo and Addis Ababa before being recruited by the CDC. "If I had my druthers," says McDade, "I think I'd like to be a teacher. Unfortunately, rickettsia is a very low-supply, low-demand field. There are very few positions for teaching the subject; med students in the U.S. may have only one lecture on the subject." Economics thus conspired to put Shepherd and McDade together at a time when the hunt for a Legionnaires' disease organism was flagging badly.

Fraser's report referred to an elevation of SGOT, an enzyme, in the victims. Higher amounts of SGOT may presage liver damage, one of the signs of rickettsial diseases. Furthermore, one theory had suggested Legionnaires' disease was a form of Q fever, a rickettsial illness.

McDade was dubious at first. "Rickettsiae, with the exception of Q fever, are carried by arthropods [a genus of insects]. Q fever is transmitted by rats. Nobody said anything about an increase in the Philadelphia rat population. Q fever usually has a very low fatality rate. The disease is usually seen in conjunction with domestic animals, in contaminated milk. It's not typically found in epidemic form."

Even though none of this fitted the Legionnaires' disease picture, McDade decided to look again for rickettsiae and any other abnormalities. He describes the process as "looking for a contact lens all over a basketball court with your eyes four inches from the floor."

It was only several hours into his first examination that McDade noticed something different, a collection of bright-red, almost sausagelike shapes amid the purplish blob of a spleen cell. Back in August when he had first looked for rickettsiae, McDade had seen a few of these, but he had assumed then that these were a typical bacterial contaminant that flowers upon death.

He summoned Shepherd for an inspection. "I didn't tell him what kinds of slides I was looking at," says McDade. "I didn't want to prejudice his thinking. At the time I was also working on a project trying to find some rickettsiae from Costa Rica that were responsible for Rocky Mountain spotted fever. So Shepherd had no idea of what I was actually looking at, but he agreed that I might well be on to something. Of course I then told him that the slides were for Legionnaires' and we agreed that I should pursue the investigation."

Finding a peculiar clump of red organisms in one of the millions of cells of a victim proves nothing. To make a case against any suspect, tissue that contains the agent must be planted in a living medium where it grows and produces sickness. Back in August, McDade had injected some guinea pigs with specimens from sick Legionnaires. The animals had become feverish and died within thirty-six hours. "Ordinarily," says McDade, "there's a long incubation for rickettsiae. When those guinea pigs became febrile so quickly, we altered our routine. The rapidity of the infection suggested the presence of either bacteria or a toxic substance."

Shepherd explains further: "When we autopsied the guinea pigs we found abscesses, pus and adhesions covering the spleen, intestines, and liver. You don't get adhesions like that with Q fever. It was a thick coating, more like you'd get from a bacterial contamination. That makes you suspect a bacterial invasion that developed after the human patient died. The postmortem invasion by gut bacteria will spread and grow anywhere."

Because of the wild growth of bacteria in the guinea pigs, McDade and Shepherd in August tried a second time to inoculate guinea pigs with material from the victims of Legionnaires' disease. But on this occasion the animals were also given antibiotics calculated to suppress any bacterial contaminants. The result was that the animals remained healthy, and the conclusion was that whatever had infected the Legionnaires was not rickettsia.

Now, about four months later, McDade and Shepherd considered the sausagelike rods they had seen. "It was Christmas vacation time," says Shepherd, "a period when things kind of let up and you have some leisure to think. We gradually developed the idea that it was not a standard organism and therefore, after looking at it in smears [the tissue slides], we'd try to cultivate it and see what it does."

McDade elected to switch from guinea pigs to chicken egg yolk sacs, a common medium for rickettsial cultures. He wanted to experiment with cells free of bacterial contaminants and without an antibiotic that might interfere with an organism's growth. After several unsuccessful experiments, he requisitioned eggs from special flocks of chickens whose feed had not been dosed with antibiotics. On December 30, 1976, McDade poked needles through the shells to inject the yolk sacs, then went home to await developments.

He was hardly confident that he was on the verge of a great discovery, nor did he feel any urgency. Remembers McDade, "I didn't feel pressure. I was aware that Legionnaires' was an ongoing problem but the CDC brass was not on my tail."

In this determined but restrained atmosphere, he carried on his experiments. Each day he examined the inoculated eggs over a light, looking to see whether the embryonic chicks were still healthy.

Six days after the injections, the embryos began to die off. And by January 6, almost all had succumbed. Microscopic inspection showed swarms of the sausagelike rods infesting the yolk sacs. McDade immediately informed Shepherd and some associates in the lab. "My pulse quickened. But there's a long interval between finding an organism growing and finding it the cause of an epidemic."

It was still quite conceivable that some other organism had penetrated McDade's *cordon sanitaire* or that a germ other than the sausagelike rod had been lurking in the specimens used to inoculate the yolk sacs.

There was a much surer test. Preserved in the CDC are 250,000 vials of serum from children inoculated with the very first batch of Salk vaccine, from encephalitis outbreaks in Texas, from malaria, from victims of innumerable epidemics. In some cases the disease is unknown; in others the agent remains a mystery. The deposits in the CDC serum bank are stocked in home-style freezers and classified not only by disease but also age, sex, physical condition, and geography.

The sera contain antibodies manufactured by the hosts to ward off disease. These antibodies will react if put together again with the original malady. In the warehouse of sera lay vials of blood drawn from victims of Legionnaires' disease. McDade secured four samples and commenced a series of critical tests.

He did not reveal what he was doing to anyone other than Shepherd. Both men were well aware of the many false starts on Legionnaires' disease and desperately wanted to avoid another. They were also wary of the complications of premature publicity.

To test antibody reaction, McDade used a procedure called an indirect fluorescent antibody test (IFA). If the antibodies reacted to the bacteria in the chick embryos they would fluoresce with a unique illumination under ultraviolet light.

At about 4:00 on January 7, McDade was ready. He and Shepherd snapped off the overhead lights, switched on the ultraviolet, and took turns peering at the slides under the microscope. They saw amorphous green shapes flare under the ultraviolet. It was the hoped-for antibody reaction. No hats were flung in the air, nobody cried hurrah. Instead, McDade methodically tested three more samples from the CDC cache of serum. Only one responded under the fluorescent light. Two out of four was not conclusive evidence.

McDade pursued the study further. Blood samples from Legionnaires' disease also existed in pairs, with one specimen drawn shortly after the onset of the disease, when the patient was suffering acute symptoms, and then a second time during convalescence. In this latter stage, there are more antibodies present, as the body has mobilized a full-scale defense.

McDade and two associates, microbiologist Martha Redus and Dr. Verne Newhouse, secured five paired specimens. In theory, the sample taken during convalescence with its higher level of antibodies should produce a stronger reaction in an IFA test. McDade had left the shop and gone home when Martha Redus telephoned that night to report that in two of the five cases the results had been a steep rise in antibody level reaction.

It again was inconclusive, but suggested that the researchers were on the right track. Why all five specimens failed to react according to theory is one of the age-old mysteries about antibodies. Still, the question remained: Were the bright-red rods specific to Legionnaires' disease? Would, for example, viral pneumonia antibodies demonstrate a similar reaction?

McDade and Shepherd requisitioned sera for viral pneumonia, psittacosis, and rickettsial diseases from the CDC's specimen bank. They inoculated these samples with chick embryo cultures of the suspected agent. The tests for all these organisms were negative. Only the sausagelike rods would trigger antibodies in the cells from victims of Legionnaires' disease.

Many more samples from Legionnaires' disease victims underwent the same painstaking scrutiny. "It's a matter of pyramiding," explains Shepherd. "Once it started to go, it all fit so nicely. I would do my jogging at five in the afternoon, eat supper, and then check with Martha Redus on the fluorescent antibody tests. Everything continued to click."

The case against the fat red sausagelike rods became increasingly strong. The telltale fluorescence registered for both those Legionnaires who had been sick and in the Bellevue Stratford and for those people who had never entered the hotel but still came down with the disease, the 38 individuals who had come within a block of the hotel and were known as the Broad Street pneumonias.

McDade and Shepherd now had accumulated a lot of evidence to identify the guilty agent. Why hadn't they spotted the killer back in August? "With known organisms," explains Shepherd, "people can pull out a diagnosis easily and swiftly.

It fits a standard pattern. We know what will happen. We were looking for those standard patterns with Legionnaires' but nothing came out."

McDade puts more succinctly the problem of a microbiologist pouring over the teeming bacteria that can occupy a single slide. "If you're looking for rickettsiae, you either find rickettsiae or you don't. You don't see anything else."

About two weeks into January, David Fraser was told to be at Sencer's office in half an hour, that something "hot" had come up. "When I got there," recalls Fraser, "I saw Shep, a guy in wire-rimmed glasses whom I didn't know [McDade], and Sencer. Shepherd did the talking; he's a very careful guy and he gave a pretty tight scientific presentation of what they had accomplished without claiming positive identification of the cause of Legionnaires'. But I was convinced; it was wonderful and they'd kept their work so secret that even I had no suspicion they were on to anything."

In the following few days, McDade and Shepherd turned their attention to some unsolved mysteries in the CDC serum bank. One memorable epidemic was a 1965 onslaught at St. Elizabeth's Hospital in Washington, D.C., where ninety-four mentally handicapped patients had developed pneumonialike symptoms and sixteen had died. Says Fraser, "John Bennett [then director of the CDC's Bacterial Diseases Division] told me early in September that when we found the agent for Legionnaires' disease we would have the cause for the epidemic at St. Elizabeth's." When McDade and Shepherd took sera of the St. Elizabeth's victims from the CDC specimen cache and subjected it to the fluorescent test, Bennett was proved a prophet.

Another puzzle was a 1968 illness that had ravaged 144 persons who either visited or worked in a state office building at Pontiac, Michigan. "Pontiac fever was well known at the center," says Fraser, "but we didn't think it was related to Legionnaires' for three reasons. First of all, the severity of the illness in Pontiac was much less. There were no deaths. No one even got pneumonia. Second, the incubation period was from five to sixty-six hours. In Philadelphia, it was anywhere from two to ten days. Finally, the attack rate in Pontiac was 95 percent; almost everyone who entered that building got the disease. But the attack rate in Philadelphia was only about 5 percent." To the surprise of Fraser and others, however, tests of Pontiac fever were also positive; another medical mystery was solved. The Pontiac phenomenon also indicated that Legionnaires' disease could come in milder forms.

The discovery could no longer be kept a secret. "We figured," says Shepherd, "that within two or three weeks the news would leak out. It would have been nice to have a couple more weeks to study the matter. When you can't lose a single day, there's always the possibility that you haven't considered some other possible explanation."

Identifying the killer organism left the job of finding the best drug to combat it. The CDC assigned Dr. Vester Lewis to the task. "They picked me," says Lewis, "because there aren't too many microbiologists who have had the experience of growing organisms in embrionated eggs, working with yolk sacs." It was necessary to use eggs infected with legionella, as the bacterium was named, because at the time no one had been able to grow it in any other medium.

"After I obtained the strange organism from McDade, we got all of the antibiotics that might work," says Lewis. "I got rifampin [a drug used for leprosy] from Shepherd, tetracycline from someone else. I had prescriptions written for others, walked over to the Emory Pharmacy [Emory University is almost next door to the CDC, and the medical school includes a pharmacy] and bought the rest of the items."

Testing each antibiotic required about a week and 160 eggs. Lewis's efforts were aimed at determining what drugs in what amounts were most effective in conferring immunity against infection and in curing the disease. Rifampin and erythromycin scored the best results.

The CDC labs turned their attention to the next priority, a better way to culture legionella than infecting fertilized eggs, a way that would allow scientists to study the organism more thoroughly. In still another laboratory at the CDC, Dr. Robert Weaver experimented with various media and eventually, using an enriched agar (a gelatinous substance manufactured from seaweed), produced an abundant crop.

McDade and Shepherd meanwhile continued to study legionella. "I initially had some uneasiness about working with the materials," says McDade. "I was then new to the CDC.

This was an unknown pathogen, and in my previous work I had not spent a lot of time dealing with autopsy specimens." By the summer of 1977, McDade was more comfortable with his assignment, and at that moment disaster struck.

George Flowers and Robert Lee Dubington were employed in the lab doing custodial duties, removing equipment to be sterilized in an autoclave and bringing back sanitized glass utensils. Both men became sick on the same day. They had chills, nausea, vomiting. Their temperatures soared to 104°, and both became so weak they could not leave their beds. Within five days Flowers and Dubington were both dead.

It was hard not to fear that somehow legionella had escaped from carefully sequestered specimens. All work in the lab remained suspended until the cause of the deaths could be determined. It took several days before technicians reported tests for legionella on the victims were negative.

"We did tissue specimens," says McDade. "These can take from three days to two weeks to incubate. Eventually the cultures showed it was Rocky Mountain spotted fever."

No one yet knows how the men contracted that disease. In thirty years of CDC operations before this accident, there had been twelve infections traceable to a lab mishap, but no deaths. "Most lab infections are aerosols," says Shepherd. "It used to be quite common, but new equipment has reduced accidents considerably."

CDC personnel always protect themselves by wearing rubber gloves that insert into sealed glass cabinets containing the malevolent organisms. In the Maximum Containment Lab, where they work with the deadliest specimens, scientists wear astronaut-like space suits. Antigerm ultraviolet rays, disposable clothing, and special showers and plumbing facilities further reduce the threat of infection.

Identifying the bacterium answered one question, but several others remained. Why hadn't employees of the Bellevue Stratford gotten sick? Why had the organism suddenly appeared in Philadelphia? What was the mechanism by which the disease made its attack? How widespread was it?

CDC investigators obtained blood samples from people who had worked at the Bellevue Stratford at the time of the epidemic. The telltale green fluorescent blotches showed in tests of nearly a dozen of the staff, although none had come down with Legionnaires' disease in the summer of 1976. At some time prior to the epidemic they had probably felt ill, thought they had a light touch of the flu, and recovered without incident. The infection had rendered them immune when the deadly eruption occurred.

About the same time as the former employees were examined, a Coloradoan named Merton Smith telephoned the CDC to report that in 1974 he had attended an Odd Fellow convention at the Bellevue Stratford. Smith and a number of his brethren had become ill. When the CDC tracked down half a dozen of these Odd Fellows, IFA tests revealed an old Legionnaires' infection. Legionella had resided at the hotel for a long time.

The most significant clue to the question of how the disease spreads came after a brushfire of legionella epidemics. One of them was at the University of Indiana, where a very high percentage of the victims had spent an evening at the university's Memorial Union building. Tests of soil and water in the vicinity found colonies of legionella in neighboring streams and the Memorial Union's air-conditioning system. Even more revelatory, water samples preserved for nine years from the air conditioner at Pontiac showed the bacterium.

More interesting, just a few miles from the CDC's Atlanta headquarters, at the Lakeside Country Club, eight members came down with Legionnaires' disease in the summer of 1978. All of them played golf, but club members who restricted themselves to swimming, tennis, or just eating were not stricken.

The implication was that legionella was in the soil of the golf course. But samples of the earth failed to contain the bacterium.

"I had one of the EIS officers on the case take me out to the country club," says Fraser. "We went through the place and by sheer serendipity came across a room that had not been open when others examined the place. Inside we found a maintenance man working on the evaporative condenser for the air-conditioning system. It vented right by the tenth and sixteenth tees. We took samples of the water from the machinery and found legionella."

Legionnaires' disease also appeared at Wadsworth Medical Center in California. Cultures done on the water of the cooling towers for the Wadsworth air-conditioning system indicated the presence of the bacterium. Subsequently, tower waters had been hyperchlorinated. But Wadsworth continued to have sporadic infections of Legionnaires' disease. When Kathy Shands, a young woman in her first year at the CDC, arrived for a two-month stay, it was obvious that legionella was on a tear.

"In England they'd discovered the bacterium in a shower head," says Shands. "The first thing I did was to look there. We set up control groups to match their exposure to those of the people who became sick, but the use of showers showed no pattern. We went to talk to the engineers about how water was distributed through the hospital. We didn't seem to be getting anywhere until one engineer mentioned that in early March, people had complained that the water was black. 'Black? What do you mean?' I asked.

"They explained that the place had an emergency water system. If water pressure in the hospital dropped, a pump was activated automatically. By means of a separate tank in the main building, the pump would provide water as high as the sixth floor.

"During a test the normal water system was shut down, but the emergency pump failed to work. Engineers quickly reopened pipes to restore the regular system. It was then that the brown and black water came out of the faucets.

"We found a wing of the hospital that contained no patients," says Shands, "and then deliberately had engineers reduce the pressure. The water samples we tested came out a cloudy brown, as if they had many organisms. When hyperchlorinated, the water cleared. We couldn't find direct evidence; everybody drank water, some took hot showers, some cold, and there was no clear pattern for the infection. But the circumstantial evidence pointed to water from the emergency supply as the breeding grounds for the disease."

Research on the Legionnaires' disease front is quiet now. The bacterium has apparently been around for a considerable period of time. Fortunately, it is not one of the more robust forms of life. It may be held in check by other bacteria competing for a place to grow. It may lie in the ground for long periods of time only to spring to life during an upheaval from construction or some natural disturbance. Hurled into the air in the fine dust, the bacterium comes to rest in the hospitable temperatures of air-conditioning pools or groundwater.

There was, according to Fraser, remarkably little construction in downtown Philadelphia that summer of 1976. But somehow legionella in the tepid waters of the Bellevue Stratford cooling towers began to colonize, doubling their numbers every six hours. As the huge fans of the air conditioner labored to cool the conventioneers, water from the cooling towers ran down the side of the building. Nature sought to protect humans; the sun's ultraviolet rays probably killed many of the bacteria. But some of the water reached the street as a mist so fine it was undetected by passersby. The vapors infected people who came within a block of the hotel. Much of the lethal mix was then sucked back into the intake vents that distributed air to the lobby of the hotel. There, hundreds of Legionnaires breathed in the germs. That's a partial explanation. Fraser notes that people who drank water were more likely to be sick, and how legionella made its way into the potable water is unknown. The other unanswered question is why the bacteria chose to bloom at the moment it did.

Legionella varies in its attack rate and its virulence. That's explained by different strains of the bacterium and by the population victimized. A high proportion of the Philadelphia dead had underlying conditions, advanced age, cardiovascular problems. Cigarette smoking added considerably to the risk of death. The disease showed a propensity for hospitals, where people are already debilitated.

For the time being, legionella is suppressed through the simple treatment of cooling-tower pools with chlorine. "At least half the air-conditioning systems we tested," says Fraser, "showed evidence of legionella." On the other hand, the bacterium is now described as "ubiquitous" in distribution. Equally disquieting, M. A. Horowitz, an EIS alumnus, and S. C. Silverstein of Rockefeller University have demonstrated that legionella can survive and multiply within human blood macrophages, the large cells that destroy such invaders.

At least seven varieties of legionella have been identified since McDade's discovery. The CDC estimates that from 50,000 to 70,000 Americans contract some form of Legionnaires' disease annually with as many as 3,000 deaths.

The various members of the original Legionnaires' disease task force have gone off to other endeavors. Walter Orenstein returned to the measles program, which, with mandated vaccination of schoolchildren, seems on the verge of wiping out endemic measles. David Heymann spent time in Africa combating the sinister hemorrhagic fevers which once were suspected of causing the Philadelphia epidemic, and then was assigned to an antimalarial project. Kathy Shands returned from the Wadsworth Hospital investigation to lead the task force on toxic shock syndrome.

The laboratory scientists busied themselves with more arcane research. Shepherd focused his attention on leprosy and the disease's growing resistance to dapsone, the preferred drug remedy. McDade was endowed with the dubious form of immortality peculiar to the medical profession when in honor of his efforts a strain of Legionnaires' disease, previously listed as Tatlock or Pittsburgh pneumonia, was redesignated *Legionella McDadiensis*. Actually, there had been some suggestion that he lend his name to the entire genus of bacteria. "The decision is usually something colleagues make," says McDade, "and I respectfully declined. I felt a little funny about having it named for me. Besides, there were a great number of people who worked on the project." In the lab McDade shifted his attention to a genuine rickettsial disease, typhus.

Sharrar has been promoted to the job of director of the Communicable Diseases Control Division of the Philadelphia Health Department. More than five years after the epidemic, he mused, "I have mixed feelings. It was an exciting challenge from an epidemiological standpoint, medically dramatic. But I feel frustrated that we didn't get the complete answers on the outbreak. We still don't really know where the disease came from. We can't even prove that it was directly connected to the hotel. I sometimes wish I could be faced with another outbreak of disease, knowing what I know now. There are things we might have done . . ." His voice trails off.

David Sencer, who was director of the CDC during the epidemic and the period in which the major investigative work was done, lost his job. The Carter administration, which took power in 1977, dumped Sencer most obviously because the swine flu immunization program he favored proved a fiasco and possibly because of lingering doubts about the handling of the initial phases of the epidemic.

An extraordinary reincarnation has occurred at the ill-fated hotel. Investors purchased the Fairmount and re-christened it the Bellevue Stratford. When Sharrar's twin brother was married in Philadelphia, family members were put up at the Bellevue Stratford. "It's a perfectly safe building," says Robert Sharrar, who still routinely passes it on the way to work.

David Fraser quietly works for the CDC in Washington, D.C. In the intervening years he has visited Egypt frequently on a program to combat streptococcal infections and has worked on studies of leprosy. "I thought my excitement in my career peaked when I was involved in a Lassa fever outbreak in Sierra Leone," says Fraser. "Then came Legionnaires'. I doubt if anything will ever match that."

In the remarks of Sharrar and Fraser, as for many epidemiologists, there is an almost universal regret. Those who hunted legionella recognize that like Sherlock Holmes, never again will they face so worthy, albeit so treacherously evil, an adversary as Dr. Moriarty.

The John Snow Disease

CHOLERA. It runs "so rapid a course that a man in good health at daybreak may be dead and buried at nightfall." So wrote a scholar of the greatest health scourge of the past two centuries.

Cholera broke out of its birthplace, India, in the early 1800s, following British troops westward and sailing east aboard merchant ships. The first pandemic killed an estimated 2 million people as it ravaged the Near East and parts of Russia.

The disease steadily moved across Europe, striking Paris in 1832. Poet Heinrich Heine was present the night of a masked ball and told of a harlequin who suddenly collapsed and died. In the ensuing Paris epidemic citizens expired so swiftly and in such great numbers that coffin makers could not keep up with the demand. Corpses were hauled away and buried in sacks.

By the middle of the nineteenth century, cholera was a fixture in Russia. It slaughtered a million Russians in the Fifth Pandemic, including composer Peter Tschaikovsky. Between 1846 and 1863, 54,000 cholera deaths were counted in England. There were 100,000 victims in Hungary during 1875. In Manila they died at the rate of 1,000 a day.

Steam power and rapid transportation brought to America Irish immigrants bearing Asiatic cholera. A single outburst felled 3,000 between Montreal and Quebec; thousands perished in New York City and Mexico City.

Cholera conquest knows two heroes: the great German bacteriologist Robert Koch, who isolated a *Vibrio cholerae* under a microscope in 1884; and a short-lived British doctor named John Snow.

Cholera, Snow, and the CDC have a special relationship. In 1849, the British anesthetist realized that the disease must be a waterborne infection. This was during an age when disease was regarded by many as divinely or satanically inspired or else the mark of character defects.

Five years later, during another massive outbreak in London, Snow calculated the risk of infection was far greater if a person drank water supplied by the Southwark and Vauxhall Company than if from a competitor. Snow traced the higher incidence to a single pump on Broad Street beside the Thames. He arranged for the pump handle to be removed. Cholera cases dropped dramatically.

To commemorate the achievement, the John Snow Pub now stands at the site of the old pump. Those who complete the EIS program at the CDC receive an emblem bearing a replica of a barrel of Watney's Ale, the brew dispensed at the John Snow Pub. Like pilgrims journeying to a holy site, CDC people visiting Britain frequently call at the John Snow.

Cholera no longer menaces large numbers of people in highly developed countries with pure water supplies and good sanitation. Still, tens of thousands of cases occur annually in some parts of the world. In the United States prior to George Charpentier's illness, the last recorded cholera infection had been at Port Lavaca, Texas, in 1973. The very rareness of cholera in this country makes it all the more dangerous for any person who develops it, because a doctor is unlikely to think of cholera. Undiagnosed and untreated, cholera kills one out of every two people it strikes.

The spiritual descendant of John Snow assigned to find the source of Charpentier's illness was Dr. Paul Blake. A soft-spoken, reserved man in his late-30s, Blake spent the first ten years of his life living in Angola, where his parents were missionaries. "I suppose I became interested in medicine," says Blake, "when I had some problems as a kid, nonmalignant tumors. I was influenced by the doctor who treated me."

He started his medical career with a strong interest in parasitic diseases and served his EIS time in Puerto Rico. The CDC chose him for a career-development program, and Blake studied at Harvard's School of Public Health. "Shortly after I returned to Atlanta in 1974," says Blake, "there was an outbreak of cholera in Portugal. I happen to speak Portuguese [a carryover from those years in Angola], so I was sent." The experience grew into a professional absorption with the genus of bacteria that includes the organisms responsible for cholera.

Charpentier's sickness posed some hard questions for Blake. "We discovered the cholera really by accident. Very few hospitals would have gone on to use the appropriate test. It's a special one, costs maybe an extra $25, and the possibility is so remote. But going back to Port Lavaca and now Charpentier, we had to ask ourselves whether cholera is endemic to the United States. We also had to consider whether the organism might have come from a ship that had been in a foreign port and discharged it in a way that Charpentier could have ingested it."

The suspected territory, southwestern Louisiana, stands like a foot on the Gulf of Mexico with the toes reaching out to touch Texas. Flat, lowland country, only a few feet above sea level, the marshy ground extends as much as 25 miles toward the interior of the state. Near the coast the water turns salty, but it freshens inland. Lakes dot the marsh, and ship canals provide access for oceangoing vessels that voyage as far as Lake Charles.

The ethnic background of the residents is French. Many of these Cajuns, particularly the older ones, speak very little English. There is even a hint of Gaul in the southern burr of George Charpentier. Adding to the mix are some 150 refugees from Vietnam who settled in the area in 1975. To some, these newcomers from the Far East seemed a likely source of cholera.

The entire parish of Vermillion includes only 50,000 people, and about a quarter of these live in the principal city, Abbeville. Vermillion Parish's economy depends largely on oil, and offshore rigs dot the landscape. A second resource is seafood—shrimp and crab.

When Paul Blake arrived in Abbeville, it was several weeks after the desperately ill Charpentier had been admitted to the hospital. The oil driller had been slowly nursed back to health, thanks to huge infusions of intravenous fluids and massive doses of antibiotics. "I don't think I would have lived if they hadn't treated me," says Charpentier. "When they started that intravenous it was only thirty minutes before I would lose it. Without the drugs and more of the intravenous I would have died."

Blake's first step was a visit to Charpentier. "The family, Charpentier and his wife and a daughter, lived in a middle-class, scrupulously clean home on the outskirts of Abbeville," says Blake. "Their drinking water came from a well in the backyard. Sewage from the house fed into a septic tank about 40 feet from the well, and the effluent from the tank ran into an open ditch that drained into the nearby Vermillion River. Considering the distance between the two systems, it was un-likely that sewage could have contaminated the family drink-ing water."

Blake questioned Charpentier about his diet in the days immediately preceding his illness. Charpentier had eaten and drunk only at his home or that of a friend. He had not eaten any raw seafoods, the most common source of cholera. He had, however, dined on cooked seafood—shrimp and eggplant casserole, boiled shrimp and crabs, and fried shrimp and crabs.

On August 7, Charpentier, whose work schedule was seven days on a rig and seven days of free time, had spent the day at the nearby Rockefeller Wildlife Refuge catching shrimp and crabs from a canal. He carefully avoided eating the sea-food raw, and he was equally prudent in avoiding contamina-tion of the food and drink he toted with him.

Charpentier packed the crabs and shrimp in an ice-filled chest and carried the delicacies home. That evening he boiled some of the shrimp. "You can only boil them for seven minutes," advises Charpentier. "If you boil them for ten min-utes or more you can't peel them." The blue crabs, beauties measuring as much as 7 inches from tip to tip, Charpentier cooked for an estimated twenty minutes. While the seafood was cooking, the chest in which the food had been stored was washed with a detergent and water. When Blake examined it, he noticed some punctures and bubbles in the plastic shell. Conceivably, these would have allowed the retention of any contaminated water from the marsh or the seafood. And after the crabs had been cooked they were stored briefly in the chest.

The family and two guests had feasted on the boiled shrimp and crab. Part of the day's catch was cleaned and frozen, while the remainder was dipped in batter and deep-fried and provided lunch the following day.

The only person who had come down with cholera was Charpentier; none of those who shared his meals became sick, nor did their blood reveal antibody levels suggesting a vibrio attack. "We didn't find any *Vibrio cholerae* in samples drawn from the family's water well, the septic tank, or the commercially produced ice used by Charpentier," notes Blake. "We tested the ten packages of frozen raw shrimp and a package of raw cleaned crabs left from an earlier catch at the refuge. These were all negative for *vibrio cholerae*."

Blake then traveled with Charpentier on an excursion into the Rockefeller preserve. "The site where he had caught the shrimp and crabs," recalls Blake, "was a good 13 miles from the nearest town and actually 25 miles from any community that might have drained sewage into the place. There were always three to fifteen cars parked in the vicinity, and an occasional bus came along. There were no sanitary facilities and considerable evidence of what might be called promiscuous defecation."

"Blake threw out a couple of nets trying to catch some crabs or shrimp," remembers Charpentier, "but he didn't get much." Charpentier himself was not very eager to fish, thanks to his memories of his ordeal. "I didn't eat any seafood for a year," says Charpentier.

Blake's main purpose in visiting the area was to collect water specimens that could be tested for the presence of vibrios. He also placed ten Moore swabs (Y-shaped wads of gauze wrapped around a wire armature) in the canal for two hours. The swabs, which soak up water, are a means of detecting the presence of bacterial agents.

Blake was also extremely curious to learn if other cases of cholera had, as Charpentier's almost did, escaped detection. "We went back into the hospital records for two years," says Blake, "looking for bacterial infections, gastroenteritis, colitis, viral intestinal infections, and parasitic intestinal infections; anyone with a severe disease also marked by low blood pressure. In two people who fitted the syndrome we found elevated levels of cholera antibodies."

The CDC investigator, in cooperation with state and local agencies, arranged a much wider stakeout to ensure no new cases of cholera escaped notice. Trolling for vibrios with Moore swabs was extended to many points in local sewage systems.

The intensified watch paid off in a few weeks. Alerted to the possibility of cholera, hospitals routinely performed the appropriate tests and diagnosed three new patients. One of these was a woman who arrived at the hospital emergency room with no detectable blood pressure. It took a massive life-support effort to save her. She survived only through huge amounts of intravenous feedings and copious antibiotics. At one point her kidneys quit working and she received treatment on a dialysis machine. Like Charpentier, she became sick after a meal of cooked crabs, although the catch occurred a good 20 miles from where Charpentier cast his nets.

Nine days later the hospital in Lafayette reported a cholera patient. "She also had eaten cooked crab," says Blake. "The seafood was from White Lake, a body of water in the marshes. The crabs were bought from a fisherman, boiled, and then served to the patient, her husband, and three guests."

Blake ferreted out every person who had partaken of the White Lake crab catch. He discovered a total of four more cases of cholera infection. Moore swabs picked up some vibrios in communities other than Abbeville, and a block-by-block survey of that city found several more people, who appeared to have played host to vibrios.

Altogether, Blake and his associates confirmed that eleven people, starting with Charpentier, had contracted cholera in the late summer of 1978. "It became front-page news in the area," says Blake, "and the story was on TV every day. There was no panic, but the people were a little surprised to see us so concerned about the disease. That in turn made them worry about the long-term possibilities."

"I was shocked when they told me what it was," says Charpentier. "You read about something like that, you don't have any idea that you could ever get it."

"I have a healthy respect for cholera myself," says Blake. "But I'd rather have cholera than typhoid, shigella, typhus, or some other infections. We know very well how to treat cholera [with antibiotics and replenishment of lost body fluids] once it is diagnosed. It is true that someone can die in a day from cholera, but the disease covers a gamut of severity.

It can be mild, almost unnoticeable, all the way to life-threatening. There are so few cases in the United States that you don't usually see the extreme sickness."

There are some known risk factors associated with cholera. Stomach operations may leave a site favorable to vibrios, although none of Blake's eleven cases reported any gastric surgery. Travel to some parts of the world exposes to cholera, and visitors to those areas can be inoculated against the disease. None of the people in Louisiana, however, had even left their state.

None used antacids, which is another important point in cholera infections. Stomach acidity provides protection against cholera. In a research project conducted by Dr. Robert Hornick and co-workers at the University of Maryland School of Medicine, volunteers from the state prison drank water laced with varying amounts of vibrios. Hornick found that when a buffering agent was swallowed with the contaminated water, susceptibility to infection rose significantly.

If Blake hoped to explain how Carpentier and the other ten cases caught cholera he would have to find the source of the vibrios. One popular hypothesis was the newly settled refugees from Vietnam might have brought cholera with them.

However, the germs isolated in Louisiana and at Port Lavaca, Texas, were not characteristic of the Far Eastern strain of cholera.

"Some bacteria have been known in our lab experiments," says Blake, "to go from Inaba [along the Arabian coast] to Ogawa [in the Far East], but that kind of shift does not readily occur in humans or in their environment. We certainly could not see any signs of this change in Louisiana."

Blake kept coming back to the one element common in all eleven victims, consumption of crabs. But in every case the boiling or steaming would have destroyed the vibrios.

"In Italy," notes Blake, "raw mussels are contaminated by the practice of freshening them with polluted bay water while they're on sale. In Portugal, the cockles were eaten raw or only partially cooked. They'd been harvested from beds polluted with local sewage. In the Gilbert Islands and Guam, similar situations occurred." Some contaminated water reached the Louisiana marshes, but nowhere near what had been seen at the sites of cholera outbreaks in other countries. "However,

it does not take many cases to infect a fairly large area,"
observes Blake. "We projected that a single patient could infect a body of water 2,500 square kilometers in area to a
depth of one meter." The reason is the fecundity of vibrios.
A single one that manages to crash through the stomach's
gastric-acid barrier will multiply in astronomical figures in the
rich mix of the human gut.

Blake found an explanation for the Louisiana phenomenon
in some of the literature on the disease. "Until 1978," says he,
"I thought cholera required passage through a human intestine
before it could grow. I taught people that if you could just
keep sewage away from food, you could break the cholera
cycle." The earlier outbreaks in Italy, Portugal, and the South
Pacific all seemed to bear this out. But the eleven cases in
Louisiana did not fit this pattern.

However, Blake came across an ancient report by Japanese
scientists to the League of Nations which claimed that cholera
could multiply in food as well as in the fertile soil of the
human intestine. Even more startling was a paper by Ross
Sutton, an Australian epidemiologist, who cracked the mystery of a cholera epidemic that ravaged forty-seven passengers
on a jet aircraft. Sutton deduced that the travelers were infected by a cooked stuffed-egg concoction that became a
reservoir teeming with vibrios. Sutton, in fact, managed to
grow cholera in the hors d'oeuvres at a laboratory.

Blake realized that the cholera vibrios might have invaded
the crabs themselves. "We began to try to recover vibrios
from the seafood and the environment from which it came,"
says Blake. The search was only partially successful. None of
the crabs captured by the scientists contained the organism,
although one shrimp from a canal did. Moore swabs dropped
at two sites, however, registered positive for cholera; victims
had consumed crabs caught near these places.

The scientists ran a series of cooking tests on lab-infected
crabs. "If cooked only eight minutes or steamed for just
twenty-five," says Blake, "the crabs had a red color, looked
firm, and appeared well cooked. But they still contained
vibrios. Furthermore, we found that sometimes the crabs will
float to the surface during the cooking with their backs out of
the water; that part doesn't get as cooked." This is particularly
significant, according to Blake, because vibrios have an affinity

for chitin, the horny cartilage of the crab's back and exoskeleton. Living in the chitin that received less cooking, vibrios also are protected by that substance against the ravages of stomach acid.

"To our knowledge," remarks Blake, "this is the first time that cooked crabs have been incriminated as a means of transmitting cholera. My guess is that the crabs either just happened to have been in a localized hotbed of *Vibrio cholerae* or else some of the animals upon which crabs feed concentrated vibrios."

Cholera faded from the Louisiana consciousness until a curious episode in 1981. One September Wednesday, Robert Sargeant (pseudonym), a Cajun like Charpentier, boarded an oil rig stationed in the Intercoastal Waterway south of Port Arthur, Texas. A husky fellow, Sargeant was what's known as a shaker-hand. His job was to swab down the decks and machinery with a wide-bore hose. It is messy, dirty work. At the end of a day, Sargeant would be soaked by spray and splashes.

On a Friday night he and his mates sat down to a dinner of well-cooked seafood. A day or so later, Sargeant began to suffer diarrhea, cramps, nausea, and dizziness. He assumed he had downed "a bad oyster" and managed to stick out his seven-day tour. Back home in Louisiana he visited a doctor for his continuing stomach troubles. To be on the safe side, the physician took a stool sample and sent it in to the state health department. Meanwhile, Sargeant routinely recovered thanks to treatment with an antibiotic.

A thorough screening of the stool sample, however, established the presence of a cholera vibrio. Immediately, state epidemiologist Caraway, recalling the case of Charpentier, ordered a check on others working that oil rig (most of the employees were Louisiana citizens rather than Texans). Ultimately, investigators learned that ten men in the crew with Sargeant and eight visitors during that period all showed signs of a cholera infection.

Indeed, Dr. Jeffrey Johnston, an EIS officer posted to the Louisiana Health Department, says, "One man had passed out on the toilet at his home. He had been taken by ambulance to a hospital. In the emergency room they couldn't find any pulse. They managed to save him. Another man was also hospitalized, and four others had been to see doctors because of their condition."

The big question was the mechanism by which the infection had spread. No person aboard the rig the week before or the week after Sargeant's seven-day tour had become ill. Sargeant was the first to be sick, after eating the seafood. Although it is also possible that he ingested vibrios while working with the hose, Caraway believes he must have eaten cholera-infected seafood at the dinner.

The infection followed the classic pattern of an epidemic. For two days of Sargeant's tour, and coinciding with the onset of his diarrhea, sewage from the drilling barge was accidentally permitted to enter the fresh-water syetem used for drinking and preparing food. Once Sargeant was sick, the discharge from toilets at one end of the vessel which he used was carried by the waterway's currents to the other end, where it could mix with potable supplies. The cross-contamination had already been discovered and repaired by the time Sargeant and the other crew members completed their stints. Those who were aboard before or after Sargeant, therefore, were never exposed to contaminated drinking water.

For a man whose association with cholera is based upon the accident of speaking the Portuguese tongue, Blake is wholly committed to the subject. "The deeper you get into the area, the more you can put together. You may think that you know but you don't. You're never going to know all there is about vibrios; they're a poorly defined organism. There is *Vibrio cholerae* and there are vibrio without cholera. There are many more diseases involving vibrios than formerly believed."

He is obviously a man who relishes the pursuit of research in a laboratory far more than the role of a hands-on healer. "I thought originally I would specialize in internal medicine," says Blake. "But I suffered too much with the patients, particularly those with cancer. I'd work, work, and work, only to see them get worse and worse. So many died, and I'd feel terrible."

There is one more curious note about cholera. It is a seasonal disease. The Port Lavaca, Texas, case happened in August, the Louisiana epidemic with Charpentier in August

and September, and the oil-rig outburst at the start of autumn.
Blake came across the comments of Thomas Sydenham, the
seventeenth-century British physician credited with offering
the first modern description of cholera. Wrote Sydenham,
"This disease . . . comes as certainly at the latter end of
summer and the approach of autumn, as swallows at the beginning of spring and as cuckoos at the heat of the following
season."

According to Blake, the vibrio now has permanent residence
in Louisiana. It may not show up with the certainty of cuckoos
at the beginning of summer but, says Blake, "I would expect
to see occasional cases popping up every year or so." That
may not sound ominous, but the explosive nature of the disease, as demonstrated aboard the oil-drilling rig, suggests
vibrio still packs a dangerous punch.

CHAPTER
4

The Gay Men's Disease

SOMETHING WAS KILLING the gay men of America. The pace of assassinations was quickening, adding more and more victims, bringing swifter and swifter deaths. The murder weapons were two obscure diseases, *Pneumocystis carinii* pneumonia (PCP) and Kaposi's sarcoma (KS), a malignant tumorous growth.

Dr. James Curran, the CDC expert in charge of the investigation into the phenomenon, was stunned by his experiences. "One man in particular made an enormous impact upon me," says Curran. "In January, his lymph nodes became swollen. By march he had been diagnosed as having Kaposi's. The small, purplish spot was removed surgically; he had both radiation and chemotherapy. By July he believed he was cured.

"I saw him in his office then. He was a very dynamic individual, a man who operated with an eight-button phone. He told me he was cured, but I didn't know anyone who had been cured at the time. I didn't say anything to contradict him. In October he developed PCP, and I saw him just as he was going into an intensive-care ward. I had tears in my eyes as I saw him gasping for breath. He seemed to realize he was dying, and he managed to tell me that he thought it was all because of his life-style. In November, he died.

"It's not just the sudden sickness," remarks Curran, "but it is the fact that the publicity about the affair has tagged the victims as gay. Many of them were married men who had led separate gay lives, and now the diseases have revealed this side of them. The guilt is enormous, the dealing with parents and wives traumatic."

Curran's reaction was not unique. Dr. Alex Kelter, one of the EIS officers assigned to the project, felt much the same shock. A public health officer in the Southwest before he signed up with the CDC, Kelter's experience had been largely in the area of environmental hazards created by manufacturing and mining installations.

"The patients I saw were very well informed," says Kelter. "You could tell by the kinds of questions they asked that they were aware the problem was of growing concern to gay men. We told them everything we knew, which unfortunately was not too much." For that matter, the patients themselves could offer very little information to help explain what was happening to them.

"Almost invariably," says Kelter, "we'd be asked, 'What is the prognosis?' It was the hardest question. I tried not to give an answer because I was not in a position to give a good answer. That was more appropriate for the doctor taking care of them. And the truth is that at that point we weren't paying much attention to therapy and what could be done. There was no way for us to even have a gut feeling about therapy."

When he recalls those moments in his conversations with patients, Kelter is obviously distressed. "It was very tempting to give a reassuring or a calming answer. But what we did know about the outcomes was not very promising. If I pushed, I tended to describe the outcome gently. But there were people who flat out asked, 'Has anyone died from this?' I would have to answer, 'Yes.' Then they would invariably ask, 'How many?'

"When they questioned me like that I told them, but I made sure that I said, 'Eight out of twenty cases,' rather than just saying, 'There have been eight deaths.' It was hard, but I was not going to tell them something I knew was not true."

Physicians traditionally are supposed to be able to wall themselves off from any emotional feelings when a patient is mortally ill. Some, like cholera expert Paul Blake, admit that one of the attractions of research is that it removes them from the practice of clinical medicine, where inevitably the doctor faces the dying. CDC people rarely become intimately involved in the lives of the sick, but Curran continued to be distressed by what he saw. "I heard about a pair of brothers, both gay," says Curran. "One had already died of PCP. The other is in and out of a hospital as his condition rapidly deteriorates." Curran lifts his hands in a gesture of frustration as he mentions the case.

Nothing in Curran's background would mark him as the obvious choice to investigate PCP and KS among gays. The son of a Detroit businessman, Curran thought of a medical career while still in grammar school. After undergraduate work at Notre Dame, he attended medical school at the University of Michigan.

"When I finished I planned to specialize in gynecology with particular attention to pelvic infections," he says. "The Vietnam War was on at the time, and the military owned you once you became a doctor, however. I heard that the government was about to establish a family service health program. I applied and appeared to be accepted, but like so many proposals of this nature, it was never established. However, I was referred to the CDC, which wanted someone who was not a dermatologist for the venereal-disease unit. They took me on, and for my military obligation I worked for the CDC in Tennessee." (The war in Vietnam was a marvelously effective recruiter of good minds for the CDC.)

"I became hooked on public health," says Curran. "It was more socially oriented and it seemed you could have a greater impact than if you just treated individuals." Through the CDC, Curran did postgraduate study, earning a degree in public health at Harvard before he moved with his wife and two young children to Atlanta, where he rose to the job of deputy director of the Venereal Disease Control Division.

At his offices in Atlanta, Curran and some associates hammered out the directions of their investigation. "We found that we could concentrate in a few areas," says Curran. "Checking around, we learned that 90 percent of the cases were in New York City, Los Angeles, San Francisco, and Atlanta. Basically, there were none in Albany, Rochester, Oklahoma City, and other places."

The investigators could not hope to find patients themselves; they needed to identify physicians handling cases. "It was very difficult," recalls Kelter. "We'd hear that Dr. so-and-so had seen a case and we would call and ask to speak to the man. But the physician would tell us he referred the patient to someone else and then it would go on and on from there, very convoluted. Eventually, most of the patients saw dermatologists, but for many skin specialists it was the first of the type they'd ever seen. The average doctor—internist or GP—would never have seen a case.

"We did a quick and dirty three-day survey of five hundred men through VD clinics in San Francisco, New York, and Atlanta looking for possible leads, although admittedly there is a bias in surveying a group this way," notes Curran. "A group portrait of thirty-five homosexual men with KS or PCP or both showed a high level of schooling, a median of sixteen years of education. The men were extremely active sexually in terms of the number of different partners—the median figure was eighty-seven in the past year. More than three-quarters of the men had gonorrhea, and there was frequent use of marijuana, cocaine, and particularly inhalant sexual stimulants, amyl and butyl nitrite. The use of these inhalants or poppers correlated with the higher numbers of sex partners." The researchers distinguished the behavior of gay men from lesbians, who tend to have fewer partners and conduct relationships over longer periods of time.

"There were a lot of theories by people at the start," says Curran. "You get heterosexual doctors examining gays and they jump on the first possible hypothesis, that it must be due to the sexual behavior of homosexuals. Because gays are involved, there is also an assumption that they are doing drugs. There were suggestions that it had something to do with amebiasis, a type of dysentery that poses a particular threat to gay men because the guilty protozoa can be spread through anal contact. There wasn't any evidence for this either.

"There was no relationship established between Kaposi's and sexual preference in any medical literature," continues Curran. "The illnesses we saw were typical serious infections for immunosuppressed hosts." These include PCP, crypto-coccal meningitis (a disease of the delicate membranes that cover the brain and spinal cord), cerebral toxoplasmosis (a parasitic infection), the viruses herpes simplex and herpes zoster (the former may be the familiar cold sore or, in a different strain, the venereally transmitted virus infection; the latter is somewhat akin to chicken pox and is also known as shingles).

"I was fairly certain," said Curran early in the investigation, "that there wasn't going to be any smoking gun that would explain this breakdown in the immunosuppressive system. One theory was that some kind of immunosuppressive event triggers these kinds of infections. These kinds of infections ordinarily occurred in people with some kind of breakdown in their normal cellular immunity. Also those patients with Kaposi's who were receiving immunosuppressive therapy was stopped."

During a conversation with Alex Kelter, a patient mentioned that as a child he had had radiation treatment for a severe case of acne. "A light bulb went off in my head," recalls Kelter. "Boy, that makes a lot of sense, I thought. Questions about previous radiation hadn't been routinely asked. Then we checked with everyone else; not a single one had ever had radiation."

There was, however, one early clue, the prevalence of cytomegalovirus (CMV). The structure of this virus resembles that of a herpes simplex virus, but unlike the latter it is not necessarily a sexually transmitted agent. CMV infections run rampant among homosexual men, and CMV appears to dampen the effectiveness of the body's natural immunosuppressive apparatus. Studies of tumor structures also have indicated CMV plays an undefined role in the development of Kaposi's sarcoma. On the other hand, CMV infections are common among young heterosexual men (one estimate says that 60 to 75 percent of the population bear CMV virus in their bodies without any disease). Indeed, the recovery of Pope John Paul II from the attempt on his life was complicated by a CMV infection of unknown origins. Possibly the organisms came from blood transfusions during and after the Pope's surgery. CMV offered a thin thread but one of the few that seemed to have any strength upon which to hang an explanation.

Curran set out to discover if male homosexuality itself or the life-style of a sexually active gay results in exposures to infectious agents or substances which themselves or in combination with CMV weaken the body's immunosuppressive abilities. The consequences might be cancer or predisposition to KS and PCP.

"The scientific interest in this investigation almost outweighed the public health concerns," said Curran. "In the beginning there were at least as many if not more people studying the matter than there are known cases of PCP and KS. This may be the largest CDC investigation of recent years, at least in terms of the disciplines involved. We've got three of the centers with eight different divisions working on it plus the Epidemiology Program Office. For example, I'm from the VD Control Division in the Center for Prevention Services; there are people from the Infectious Diseases Division, and the Virology Division out of the Center for Infectious Diseases. We've got experts from the Immunology Division, which is part of the same center, and the EIS Field Services Division is under the Epidemiology Program Office." Forty people were part-time on the project, ten more spent every waking hour devoted to the hunt.

"What attracts everyone is the possibility of dramatic discoveries in the relationship of the immune system," explains Curran. "There is a theory that cancer cells exist in the bodies of most, if not all, people but the immune system keeps these cells in check. When you give a person chemotherapy that is immunosuppressive, then the cancer cells have an opportunity to develop, according to this theory. But here we have Kaposi's sarcoma. Historically, KS is evidence supporting this theory, but now the disease was occurring without any underlying condition affecting the immune system." Actually, 75 percent of the people also bear the parasite responsible for *P. carinii* pneumonia. But they don't develop PCP because of their natural resistance. Something in a handful of gay males is different.

"But you have to recognize that there's a tremendous diversity in behavior within the gay community," continues Curran. "After all, hundreds of thousands of homosexuals, young to middle-aged men, are active sexually and only a tiny fraction developed the disease. We know the disease is not genetic, or at least there's nothing to indicate that, so there must be something in the environment or life-style that combines with a certain kind of person to make specific gays vulnerable. The question is, what?

"We decided that the best way to isolate the causes was to do a thorough case-by-case study with five controls [individuals who were not sick] for every case. Two of the controls came from VD clinics, two from private and public clinics, and one was a heterosexual. One control was a friend of the victim but not a sexual partner." Age, race, sexual preference, and drug use were all part of the control mix.

"Getting private physicians to help us select controls is tricky," remarks Curran. "The doctor must be prepared to spend some time, and he can't select the first person at hand. On a random basis we may say you've got to find a gay man, 51 years old, whose last name begins with R, and who doesn't have a chronic illness. The only latitude is a range of age between 49 and 53. The physician must be aware of how to define a truly homosexual person. Ask a person if he's gay and if the man is candid he might admit, 'Oh, twenty years ago in the army, I got drunk and . . .' To some that might mean the man is gay or at least bisexual. In getting physicians and other professions to work on this study I was anxious to ensure that no obvious bias was involved. I personally interviewed all of the EIS candidates for the investigation." Among the twelve EIS officers chosen were four women.

Within the CDC, Curran discovered that there were interested professionals who either preferred to remain closet gays or to avoid any association with the project. "I received a number of unsigned notes saying, 'Have you considered thus and so?' or 'What about . . .'"

He was very circumspect in the manner of choosing controls. "When word about the project was published, we got hundreds of phone calls from gays volunteering to participate. But there's a bias built into these people. They're more likely to attempt to guess the answers to our questions. Everyone is so desperate for answers, which is natural. Gay doctors would like to think that it's a matter of drugs that they don't use. That would relieve their anxiety, but unfortunately that can't be established."

In pursuit of definitive information, Curran and the staff created documents labeled CDC Protocol #577. These included a twenty-two-page interview that covered an individual's medical history, socioeconomic background, occupational and avocational data, information on exposure to risk factors such as radiation, pets, travels, use of alcohol and drugs, medications, details on members of the family and more than three pages devoted to sexual behavior. The protocol also consisted of consent forms in which either a control or a victim agreed to provide the requested information and allowed blood and urine samples and swab samples from the inside of the mouth and the rectum.

When the matter first went public, the *New York Times* ran only a brief item, a bit surprising considering the intriguing aspects of the story. But far worse for Curran and the CDC was an account in New York City's *Village Voice*, a paper read by many gays. Columnist Alexander Cockburn accused the CDC of concocting the epidemic as a cautionary tale designed to frighten homosexuals. Cockburn sneered, "Subsequent enquiries support the view that Kaposi's Sarcoma is associated with traumatic sex, or in less elevated parlance, such activities as fist-fucking. . . ." To whom Cockburn addressed his "enquiries" (use of the British spelling and the street vernacular in a single sentence encapsulates Cockburn's style) went unrevealed, but even a rudimentary reading on the disease would have eliminated association with "traumatic sex" as absurd.

Throughout the investigation, Curran expressed mild dismay not at the way the story was played in the media, but at the absence of extensive coverage. Unwittingly, he may have explained the omission from TV shows and newspapers when he remarked, "Attitudes toward gays sometimes are subtle, like racism." And for decades the problems of nonwhites went unremarked in the newspapers unless they visited their unhappiness upon the white community. With the epidemic confined to gays and perhaps fearing that any discussion might reduce them to the level of talking about such gamy stuff as Cockburn wallowed in, the story was passed up.

Little more than six months into the hunt, Curran had confirmed 225 cases of either PCP, KS, or both among youthful gay men. Furthermore, his survey turned up a dozen or so victims with "other serious, opportunistic infections." The overall fatality rate was nearly 40 percent, an epidemiological horror surpassed only by rabies and the rare outbreaks of hemorrhagic fevers in Africa. And the figures may have been understated. Curran and his associates eliminated another sixteen cases because of the presence of a possible predisposing illness or systemic immunosuppressive therapy.

When graphed, the disease showed steadily ascending curves. By February of 1982 the CDC had received reports of seven to ten cases and two to four deaths a week. "If immunosuppression is the underlying cause of these conditions," wrote Curran in the *New England Journal of Medicine*, "then KS and PCP may represent the 'tip of the iceberg' of other conditions less readily recognized."

From the mass of data obtained through Protocol #577, Curran had separated out what he considered some of the relevant pieces to the puzzle. The oral and anal behavior of gay men substantially adds to their susceptibility to a host of infections. The way of sexual expression among gays may lead to the introduction of organisms into the intestinal tract that ordinarily never have an opportunity to settle in such fertile ground.

The rate of hepatitis B among homosexuals is high; it may spread from contaminated needles used for group drug abuse or through sexual contact. "There is also an extremely high prevalence of hepatitis B carriers among the gay population," notes Curran. Amebiasis, a parasitic infection, was also making the rounds of the homosexual community, and CMV, as Curran had learned earlier, appears to be omnipresent. These too could depress the immune response.

Another significant element was the life-style of homosexuals. "These were not closet gays," observes Curran. "They are very active sexually with a large number of different partners." Among the comparable heterosexuals the percentage of promiscuous men was considerably lower.

One more element was drug use. Dr. H. Masur and associates had reported treating eleven cases of PCP in men whose immune system appeared compromised. Six were homosexuals, but the five others, who were heterosexual, were reported to be drug abusers—heroin, methadone, alcohol, or cocaine. Laboratory studies have indicated that opiates alter cellular immunity.

Another drug, amyl nitrite, was initially believed a key factor. Small bottles with nitrites in fluid form are vended openly in the sex and head shops under such persuasive brand names as Locker Room, Bolt, Kryptonite, Head, Bullet, and Rush, among others. Those who use amyl nitrite (86.4 percent of homosexual men) claim it promises a highly sensational orgasm that seems prolonged although the feeling lasts only a moment. Curran speculated that the nitrites might play a critical role in the chain reaction leading to the two diseases. But no statistical connection could be made; this hypothesis lost credence.

"We may never find a precise answer," admits Curran, his normal intensity dimmed with a shadow of despair. "We may not tease out a single risk factor, but only a probability based upon cumulative life-style. There is no real precedent for this; scientifically it shouldn't work this way. There ought to be a correlation with the definite facts, like the chances that you'll have a blue-eyed child." But for the gay men's disease, nothing equivalent to the genes that determine the color of eyes has been discovered.

Curran worries about the lack of progress. "We may be understating the problem considerably. There are people who have had the lesion for eighteen months; all that's visible to them is a little speck on the arm, but it may be all through the man's intestinal tract. Nobody knows how to treat it; they barely are able to diagnose it. A lot of pathologists have never even seen a case. You need a biopsy to confirm it. But if you treat it with chemotherapy you wipe out what's left of the man's immune system; it leaves open the question of whether the tumor should be treated at all." Meanwhile, the rate of cases and fatalities rolls on, unabated.

"I've had to travel a lot, work hundred-hour weeks; it's difficult for my wife and kids," continues Curran. "The nature of a task force demands my time helping others maintain their energy analyzing data, doing lab work, correlating information; it's tedious stuff. The CDC is an emergency-oriented place, and it responds to that kind of pressure. Physicians are energized by an epidemic, but you can only maintain the level of enthusiasm for a period of time."

After eighteen months of investigation even the assumption that this phenomenon was something peculiar to gay men became questionable. Significantly higher rates for Kaposi's and PCP were detected among hemophiliacs (individuals with a genetic defect in their blood-clotting mechanism), among Haitians, and in drug addicts. The scientists speculated about the possibility of a viral agent again, but the answer remained well hidden.

By late 1982, the condition had received a clinical label—Acquired Immune Deficiency Syndrome (AIDS). The mystery of AIDS deepened as the CDC learned of twenty young children with the condition. They obviously could not be described as active homosexuals or drug abusers. However, in a number of cases, a member of the family was apparently either gay or a drug user.

In the winter of 1982 AIDS became a hot item for the media. Front-page stories in tabloids like the *New York Post* frightened people with an AIDS case in the family, hospital workers treating AIDS patients, guards and cops dealing with victims, and even individuals facing surgery as well as blood donors. There was confusion over transmission of the disease. The fact is, AIDS seems to be communicated only through an exchange of bodily fluids. Family members, hospital personnel, and others who have routine contact with victims do not contract AIDS. The risks from a blood transfusion are minute.

Meanwhile, Haitians protested their inclusion in the four high-risk groups, arguing that a handful of their countrymen were gay or drug users and developed AIDS as a result. The CDC researchers remained unconvinced. It calculated that 94 percent of the victims belonged to the four groups, with gays accounting for more than 70 percent of the victims.

Three years after the discovery of AIDS the CDC counted slightly more than 2,500 cases. Not a single person who lost his immunity had been reported to have regained it. However, the rate of increase slowed, possibly because gays were changing their sexual patterns or perhaps an unknown factor was limiting the spread. Gays organized protests over what they believed was inadequate financial and scientific efforts to control the epidemic. However, the CDC had 75 people full-time and 75 more part-time working on the problem, and the *Village Voice*, a paper sensitive to the gay community and often antiestablishment, defended both Jim Curran and the CDC for their dedication to the control of AIDS.

Research has focused on either a viral or fungus-like agent. The difficulty is that with the immune response destroyed, opportunistic infections can masquerade as a cause rather than be a result. The likelihood of a swift answer to AIDS is dim, but the investigation may uncover secrets about the immune system, cancer, and even the lifespan of humans.

CHAPTER
5

The Sound of Hoofbeats

PAUL COOPER ended a twenty-year hitch in the U.S. Army in 1972. As a paratrooper and a Green Beret, Cooper pulled two combat tours in Vietnam. He had been awarded a Soldier's Medal for dragging three comrades to safety from a helicopter after it crashed and was about to explode. When Glyn Caldwell first heard of Cooper, the tall, well-built former paratrooper was in the terminal stages of acute myelogenous leukemia, racked with pain as his bone marrow manufactured cells that ravaged his body. The dying man's plea for a pension for a military-service-incurred disability—blood cancer from his exposure to radiation at the nuclear test named Smokey— had already been rejected by the Veterans Administration.

Summoning his last vestiges of strength, Cooper managed to make an appearance on the ABC TV show *Good Morning America*. Among those watching was Russell Jack Dann, with his own history of dizzy spells since the days he had served with Paul Cooper at the Smokey test. One night in 1974, Dann had stepped out on the balcony of his second-floor apartment for a breath of the cool night air. Vertigo suddenly swept over him. He staggered and then tumbled backward through a rotten railing. The fall broke Dann's neck and left him a quadriplegic. Seeing and hearing his old comrade in arms Paul Cooper, Dann became convinced that the radiation he had received at Smokey was responsible for his dizziness and his subsequent ills. After several days of effort Dann managed to reach Cooper by telephone. Feeble and bedridden, Cooper extracted a tearful promise that Dann would carry the fight to the Congressional hearings on the effects of atomic tests on GIs.

When the mushroom-shaped wall of condensing water from the surrounding atmosphere and tons of dust and debris—vaporized motes packed with radioactive fission products—arose over Hiroshima in August 1945, it was a monstrous smoke signal announcing the birth of the atomic bomb. Tens of thousands of people were already dead or dying from the fury of the explosive forces and the incinerating firestorms. Thousands who escaped the initial impact of the blast or the subsequent fires would die in one to four weeks. The first symptoms would be repeated vomiting, a fever and an insatiable thirst. A few days of respite might follow, but then blood would begin to ooze from openings of the body. Hair would fall out, a deadly diarrhea would deplete them. They were all victims of radiation exposure, a problem that was to become of growing, almost obsessive concern in decades to follow.

Many Japanese who survived those first awful days after the detonation at Hiroshima may have believed the ordeal was over. But they did not understand the full effects of a nuclear explosion, the possibilities of an insidious growth of vicious diseases years later.

The process of nuclear fission, the splitting of an atom, releases an enormous amount of energy. A nuclear explosion also sheds minute components from the ruptured atom. Included may be alpha, beta, or neutron particles, and an electromagnetic stream known as gamma rays. All four are classified as ionizing radiation, meaning they bear energy.

When this ionizing radiation strikes human tissue, the energy may be sufficient to cause chemical changes in the molecules that are the building blocks of the cell. There are four possible consequences of the meeting of ionizing radiation and a cell. The radiation may simply pass through the cell without damaging it. The cell may die from the molecular reaction and be unable to reproduce itself (which is why radiation therapy is employed against cancer cells). The cell may be injured but manage to repair itself. Or it may be changed in such a way as to mutate, either immediately reproducing an abnormal version of itself or lying dormant for a number of years and then in response to some trigger mechanism—even the passage of time—multiply into a clone of cells, a malignant growth. This monstrous creation can destroy other cells and the normal functioning of organs until life can no longer be sustained. There are many versions of this disaster; they are all forms of cancer.

Medical scientists know of many things that may alter cells, turning them from industrious servants of the body into homicidal savages. Cigarette smoking is a known carcinogen. Asbestos similarly breeds cancerous growth in the respiratory cellular system. Prolonged exposure to the sun's ultraviolet rays may influence cells to malevolence. Certain viruses are capable of insinuating themselves into cells, suborning their purposes until they run amok. With age, cells may fumble their normal reproductive function, manufacturing barbarian cells that loot and pillage the working communities of the body, the vital organs. Therapeutic chemicals introduced into the system to combat diseases, including cancer, like a batch of cocktails swallowed by an unsuspecting teetotaler, may unleash hidden demons. And radiation therapies designed to diagnose conditions or to destroy malignant cells may affect innocent members of the body, like passersby who are victims in a shootout between police and criminals.

The soldiers, like Paul Cooper, who watched Smokey explode in the Nevada desert and were exposed to ionizing radiation were 40 to 50 years old and mostly civilians when Glyn Caldwell began his study of them. In the twenty years since the atomic test they could have been exposed to a number of influences on their cells, and some accounting for other risk factors than radiation at Smokey would need to be included.

On the other hand, Caldwell did possess statistics of how many cases of leukemia, thyroid cancer, heart disease, and most of the ills known to humankind that men of good health at the average age of 20 might reasonably be expected to have contracted after twenty years more of life in America. Against this template he planned to lay the experience of the witnesses to Smokey, seeing if there was something distinguishing this particular cohort of men from those who had not had the experience of exposure to an atom bomb test.

Determining whether the explosion of a nuclear bomb twenty years ago might have produced mutant, destructive cell growth after a long time lapse or whether the sick men were just the victims of the customary degeneration because of age, genetics, or other risk factors since Smokey called for a stubborn methodical mind that would not be distracted by the swirl of voices anxious to make their own points. The nominee for the investigation of Smokey, Glyn Caldwell, was a man who had already demonstrated a certain persistence of spirit in carrying out a professional career in medicine and science.

Son of a St. Louis gas station owner, Caldwell readily recalls the moment his interest in science and medicine was piqued. "My friend Herman Witte owned a microscope, and I was just fascinated by what I could see through it. Around the same time I also read Paul DeKruif's book *Microbe Hunters*. I decided that I wanted to become a GP."

Young Caldwell's ambition appeared well beyond his grasp. Family problems and troubles of his own making in high school combined to make him a ripe prospect for the military draft rather than a college education. Plucked by the army, he was shipped to Korea in 1954 to serve his time with units monitoring the uneasy truce between the two Koreas and their assorted allies. Had he remained in the States Caldwell himself might have been one of the GI guinea pigs experiencing a nuclear explosion.

After mustering out, Caldwell, in his own words, "bombed around for six months" before entering St. Louis University. He earned a Bachelor of Arts degree in 1960, but a lack of money prevented him from chasing his childhood ambition to become a physician. Instead of entering medical school, Caldwell obtained a scholarship for a graduate program at St. Louis. A thesis on viruses impressed one of Caldwell's teachers enough for him to recommend that Caldwell seek admission to medical school. "I was already married and it was tough," recalls the cancer specialist. However, he persisted and obtained a public health internship in Boston. Caldwell had never lost his interest in infectious diseases and the work of those who fought to curb them, so romantically if inaccurately described by Paul DeKruif. When an opportunity opened up at the CDC, Caldwell grabbed it. He began his career with the organization in Kansas City and then transferred to Atlanta for a series of investigations into leukemia.

"The mechanism of an epidemiological study is pretty straightforward. You try to determine whether there really is an increased morbidity [disease] or mortality incidence. It must be scientifically and accurately done. You can't depend upon reports from people who say, 'Everybody in my unit is dying.' Sometimes the data are available through review of hospital records, state and local public health agencies, or other sources. Sometimes, however, we have to collect our own information through questionnaires, interviews. And of course there must be some kind of case control, a base you can measure your findings against.

"In Smokey we had no idea of the morbidity or mortality rate among the troops present. We started to look for the ex-GIs, and that meant finding out who was there. I began with what is now the Department of Energy (DOE), which was the successor to the Atomic Energy Commission. DOE said it had no information on who was there. I tried the Department of Defense. They said they had no listing of the men at Smokey. I knew that men from the 82nd Airborne Division had been present, so I asked it for names. They told me that the units had been provisional ones, groups made up of men pulled out of different platoons, and the division had not kept a record of who served in them."

During this period, Caldwell interviewed Paul Cooper. "By now there was no doubt in Cooper's mind," says Caldwell, "that his illness was due to the exposure at Smokey. He was a very sick man, very opinionated. He had become quite bitter about all of his difficulties with the Veterans Administration, which refused to accept his illness as service-connected." The decision barred him from a 100 percent disability pension of $820 a month and benefits which would have been paid to his wife and three children following Cooper's death.

The Veterans Administration was less than enthusiastic about the search being conducted by a sister government agency. If the CDC found a significant amount of morbidity and mortality among former servicemen exposed to A-bomb tests the VA faced massive financial obligations, or at the very least a protracted series of petitions and suits to compel the VA to recognize the ill health as service-connected and its victims as eligible for pensions.

There was another sensitive aspect to the inquiry, although it was less obvious. During the 1950s, when the bulk of the nuclear-bomb tests occurred, many concerned citizens, in-

cluding a wide range of scientists, warned of potential radiation damage not only to the troops but to the rest of the nation
from fallout carried thousands of miles by air currents. A
vigorous anti-bomb campaign helped lead to a U.S.-Soviet
treaty banning above-ground nuclear explosions. Anti-nuke
forces turned their attention to the dangers alleged in nuclear
power. Interest in tracking the effects of the radiation of the
tests slacked off. The citizens of Hiroshima had been subjected
to exposures of 50 rems (units measuring radiation dosage),
while the maximum at A-bomb tests was under 5 rems and
considered highly tolerable. But if it turned out that a substantial number of men who received this low dose suffered
a significantly higher rate of cancer and other degenerative
diseases, the theories of what is a "safe" amount of radiation
would need reconsideration. That might influence thoughts of
nuclear power plants and atomic-waste disposal.

Cooper supplied Caldwell with some names of companions
at Smokey. Caldwell was still thinking in terms of several hundred men when the quest for Smokey survivors went public.
Paul Cooper and his battle with the VA for a pension (eventually granted on a technicality that did not accept the disability as connected to Smokey) had made the wire services
and the newspapers. Caldwell had also reached out for information. He wrote to the Armed Forces Radio Service and
asked it to broadcast an appeal to servicemen who might have
been at Smokey to come forward. He cooperated on production of a story in the Fort Knox, Kentucky, post newspaper,
Inside the Turret, contracted a newspaper supplement, *Parade*,
for another piece, and corresponded with Paul Jacobs, an
anti-nuclear-test, anti-nuclear-power journalist who subsequently died of cancer, possibly from having touched radioactive materials while prowling the sites of A-bomb tests.

"I started out getting maybe twenty-five letters a week from
guys who said they'd been at tests," says Caldwell. "But as
the word spread I was swamped with mail, 2,500 letters a
week. The problem was in trying to sort out who had been at
Smokey and who was at other tests."

The drumming of hoofbeats was heard by many others
besides Glyn Caldwell as he slogged after information about
the men present at Smokey. Responding to Congressional
pressure, the Defense Department had opened a hot line for

calls from those who had been involved in the tests. In the first two weeks, 10,000 calls from ex-servicemen were recorded. Claims of cancer because of exposure to nuclear radiation during atomic-bomb tests amounted to 179, and 146 others attributed different serious illnesses to the rays and particles distributed by the military's nuclear explosions. The petitioners included not only some of the estimated 250,000 to 300,000 men assigned to the postwar tests, but also some of the 4,000 troops detailed to help clean up at Hiroshima and Nagasaki after the August 1945 bombings of the two Japanese cities.

The experiences of some of the veterans of the earlier atomic age were vivid. Former marine Martin Simonis, who observed a 1955 test from a trench in the Nevada desert, said it was "like having fifty lightbulbs go off in your eyes." Some twenty years later, as a systems analyst, Simonis blamed that moment for a series of ailments—excessive calcium in his blood, a defective parathyroid gland which required four operations. "A doctor tried to find out where the devil I got something that would throw my blood off at my age. He kept asking me whether I'd gotten extensively X-rayed. . . . I told him I was at an atom-bomb blast." Simonis sought to sue the government; his stays at the hospital had cost him an average of $4,000 apiece.

O. T. Weeks as a 22-year-old airman third class was present for a series of blasts. He asserted that while stationed at Camp Desert Rock, the post where the GIs were housed, he inhaled and ingested highly radioactive particles from the explosions. His illness was not diagnosed, but Weeks complained, "I hurt twenty-four hours a day. My whole bone structure hurts." He spoke of blurred vision and a loss of equilibrium. His older daughter had defective vision and a goiter, an enlargement of her thyroid gland. If cut, she would heal with raised tissue known as keloid scars that reappeared even after cosmetic surgery. A second child exhibited motor difficulties, a third died of brain damage shortly after birth. There was no history of genetic defects in the family, insisted Weeks and his wife.

Weeks, like other veterans, had taken his case to the Veterans Administration, which refused to accept his problems as service-connected. The VA insisted the burden of proof is on the veteran, difficult to establish for a disease many years after the allegedly causal event and doubly troublesome in that Weeks's records, along with those of many other veterans, had disappeared in the 1972 fire that destroyed an estimated 17 million dossiers in the St. Louis military records storage center. VA policy required veterans to show signs of their illness either while in the service (Paul Cooper eventually was awarded a pension because his last medical records indicated enlarged lymph glands while still in the service) or within eighteen months of discharge. Since disease from radiation exposure may not surface for ten, twenty, or even thirty years, claims based on radiation were routinely rejected.

Other veterans of atomic blasts or their survivors came forward with gruesome anecdotes of health problems and complained of the VA's unyielding attitude. Russell Jack Dann described his dizziness and his accident and also told of how he had "lost teeth, my hair fell out in patches, my joints ached, and I had a low sperm count," in the first years after Smokey.

On the other hand, helicopter pilot William Dillon, who hovered a few feet above the dust-covered ground zero after the blast, reported his only health complaint was arthritis in his knees and that he was the father of two healthy kids. Another veteran of Smokey, Robert McFeeters, also announced that he, at 59, had no medical problems.

However, it was mostly a lugubrious parade of people, sick veterans, widows, and children with horrible birth defects, who lurched through the media during the late 1970s as nuclear fallout once again became a hot topic.

Glyn Caldwell's hunt might have continued to poke along, but suddenly, Congressman Tim Lee Carter of Kentucky, and a physician himself, telephoned Caldwell. The legislator reported that one of his constituents, Donald Coe, had, as a 20-year-old private, been at Smokey. Coe was now dying of what's called hairy-cell leukemia. Statistical probability indicated that in a group of men the approximate age of those at Smokey there would be perhaps two cases of leukemia. But now Caldwell was already aware of two and he had managed to locate and study the medical records of but a few hundred participants at the A-bomb blast. There was a definite sound of hoofbeats. But Caldwell did not know yet whether it was a horse or a zebra.

With the media beating the bush in search of stories like that of Paul Cooper, 500 actual participants at Smokey were flushed out for interviews by Glyn Caldwell. The CDC investigators now knew of a total of five cases of leukemia, a figure far above what might have been expected under the known incidence of that disease among a population sample this age.

The anecdotal material, however poignant, at most represented an infinitesimal percentage of those exposed. "We couldn't get to the end of the study without the publicity and the stink," remarks Caldwell, somewhat regretfully, of the furor that surrounded what he had hoped to make a dispassionate scientific survey. "But if hell hadn't been raised we might not have found the people."

His first substantial lead came with the disclosure that the Armed Forces Radiobiology Research Institute (AFRRI) had an alphabetized list of people who had been involved in atomic-weapons production or testing. "I had to badger them," says Caldwell in retrospect, "just to get the names, but there was no way of telling what events the men had been at. Then we also found out that the U. S. Army Signal Corps Depot in Lexington, Kentucky, had film badges that had been issued to people for the purposes of measuring their radiation exposure. Putting the two lists together we came up with 3,153 participants at Smokey. Now the problem was to locate them."

The exact figure actually was never firmly established. Caldwell had been aware that there were foreign observers unaccounted for, but he was surprised to learn that a former airline pilot named Clifford Keel, as a 21-year-old second lieutenant in the Tennessee National Guard, had flown a reconnaissance fighter in the vicinity of the blast. Keel was now dying of leukemia, and no one had mentioned National Guard units at Smokey.

The media attention to the investigation ignited political interest. The Subcommittee on Science and Technology of the House Committee on Commerce, under Chairman Paul Rogers, a Florida Democrat, and with Kentucky Republican Tim Lee Carter an active interrogator, convened toward the end of January 1978. (On the Senate side, a Veterans Affairs Subcommittee met later to cover the same ground.)

Caldwell feared the effects of an emotionally charged show—
"a man with an IV wheeled in on a hospital bed to testify"
—but the Congressmen were relatively restrained.

Rep. Carter questioned Caldwell closely. At one point
Carter tried to extrapolate from the body count for leukemia
(five among the first 500 histories of Smokey troops). Caldwell demurred from any speculation that the preliminary figures indicated as many as 2,500 to 3,000 leukemias among
the entire contingent of a quarter million troops that had
witnessed atomic-bomb explosions.

Russell Jack Dann, from a wheelchair, informed the subcommittee on his experience. He explained how he had been
instructed to kneel on one knee, cradle his M-1 rifle in his
arms, and shield his eyes with his hand. Like others before
him he reported that the light of the blast illuminated the
bones in his hands and fingers. "It blew my steel pot completely off. I never did find it." Dann also reported that the
trenches where he and others originally were supposed to be
stationed had caved it. The men from Dann's unit had been
trucked to an open desert area without entrenching tools that
might have enabled them to dig foxholes. Many men were
knocked sprawling in the sand from the force of the detonation.

Dann testified that when he was checked by the radiation
monitoring team, "My count was very high." The decontami-
nation measures consisted of shaking out his fatigue jacket
and brushing off his boots with a broom.

Major Alan Skerker of the Defense Nuclear Agency provided data on the monitoring of the blasts. He told the Congressmen that the entire series of tests was an operation run
by the Atomic Energy Commission but the troops and their
movements were controlled by the Department of Defense. He
testified that not only did no one keep track of the whereabouts
of the unit from the Tennessee National Guard, but also that
"no one knows who gave the order to bring them from
Tennessee."

Advised Skerker, "In Smokey, the entire radiological safety
for ground troops rested with the Sixth U. S. Army." That
organization, however, had no responsibility for anyone except army troops, which meant that U. S. Air Force participants, those from the Tennessee National Guard, and the

foreign observers, including a contingent from Canada, went unmonitored for radiation dosage.

Originally, measurements of radiation dosage were given in terms of roentgens, in honor of Wilhelm Roentgen, the German scientist who discovered X-rays in 1895. However, X-rays involve only a particular form of radiation. By international agreement a new calibration, the rad, an acronym for "radiation absorbed dose," was created. Technically a rad is 100 ergs of deposited energy per gram of matter. And if an X-ray is the source of radiation, one Roentgen equals one rad. Scientists refined their measuring tools even further in order to develop a scale specifically applicable to humans. This is the rem, or "radiation equivalent in man." It equals the amount of radiation that would produce the same biological effects as a rad of X-rays. When X-rays, which are closely akin to gamma radiation, are used, rad and rem values are equal. But since exposure to A-bombs may involve other than X-rays, the calibrations are now always done in terms of rems.

The usual method employed for measuring radiation exposure during the tests was to issue to the troops film badges about the size of a cigarette pack. Worn on the jacket or shirt, the film, encased in a light plastic cover, was sensitive to radiation and technicians could figure the number of rems a man received by the effects of the radiation upon his badge.

Originally, Caldwell had some faint hopes that he might discover an accurate set of records revealing just how much radiation individuals had received. However, as Skerker explained to the predictably appalled Congressmen, "There was no central depository" for the dosimeter records. Caldwell had access to many badges from Smokey which had been retained at Kentucky's Bluegrass Signal Corps Depot, but badges as true indices of actual exposure were highly questionable.

"Badge use was all screwed up," says Caldwell. "Some wore them for weeks, some didn't wear them at all. Many men were on hand for several tests. Some guys were simply assigned doses; if none had been recorded they gave a guy what everyone else in his outfit seemed to register." Caldwell's appraisal was borne out by the memories of men at tests.

Russell Jack Dann said that his film badge which registered radiation exposure to Smokey was collected after the test but he had no device when he observed Galileo a few days later. Former radar technician Pete Newberry, suffering from a variety of benign tumors on his body, spent six months at Camp Desert Rock, a period that included twenty-two explosions, including Smokey. But Newberry insisted the practice of the time was to change badges every two weeks, and a cumulative accounting of his exposures would have been much more than what the VA admitted. There was no badge for National Guardsmen like Cliff Keel.

Major Skerker revealed that conditions at other Nevada nuclear explosions were similarly confused. In a test shot named Nancy, film badges were not issued to individuals. "This was done," explained Skerker, "because the film dosimetry section could not keep up with the workload." One badge per platoon of twenty-five men was given out.

In the Nancy experiment, a wind shift blew radiactive materials over the trenches; fallout supposedly reached an intensity of 14 rem (5 rem was considered the maximum safe level). At the tests designated Simon and Badger, some exposures as high as 16.3 rem were recorded. In Baneberry, a modest 20-kiloton bomb exploded in a 910-foot vertical hole, a fissure opened and effluent vented to a height of 20,000 feet. Three civilians at the site died of leukemia shortly afterward.

The official documents produced at the hearings stated that the troops at Smokey were a minimum of 8 miles from ground zero when the bombs went off. But witnesses testified that the shock of the blast knocked them over; a force of that magnitude required soldiers to be considerably closer to the blast site. Other calculations placed some men at 3,000 yards, the distance Cooper and Dann claimed they were. Experts figured the amount of radiation in that area would amount to 6.3 rem of gamma radiation, 2.3 rem of neutron radiation.

Caldwell's painstakingly slow search through the files located all but about 100 of the more than 3,000 present at Smokey. There were a few individuals who refused to cooperate and would not allow their medical records to be seen, nor would they permit Caldwell to interview them. But Caldwell believes their number is too small to bias his research.

Rather than rely only on the diagnosis of attending physicians, Caldwell procured hospital clinical records of alleged leukemia patients and where feasible even obtained pathology specimens—samples of bone marrow and peripheral blood—for microscopic inspection.

The most significant finding was a sharply higher rate of leukemia, nine cases in all where the statistical expectation of the disease for this cohort should have been 3.5. The other elevated disease was in the matter of nonmelanotic skin cancer, which was double the predictable incidence.

The experience at Hiroshima and Nagasaki indicated that a higher rate of leukemia does not occur with an exposure of under 100 rems. But at Smokey the men had received an average of only 1 rem. And in spite of confusion about dosimeter readings, a special study funded by the Defense Nuclear Agency decided the error factor was no greater than two. There were, of course, the tales of the radioactive dust which the men walked through and which they breathed in. Still, Caldwell believed that this would not add greatly to the actual radiation dose. Indeed, health problems did not correlate with the available dosimeter readings. "We found twenty people with more than 5 rems, not a single leukemia in the bunch," said Caldwell.

However, the results of Smokey had to be viewed in a new light as a result of a study led by Dr. Joseph Lyon. An investigation of childhood deaths in some Utah counties in the path of fallout from the nuclear tests turned up some disquieting facts, and a single paragraph from a paper published by Lyon and associates is fraught with sinister implications. "A significant excess of leukemia deaths occurred in children up to 14 years of age living in Utah between 1959 and 1967. The excess was concentrated in the cohort of children born between 1951 and 1958, and was most pronounced in those residing in counties receiving high fallout. Over half the excess deaths (16 out of 30) occurred in the part of the state receiving the heaviest radiation exposure."

Critics of Lyon's paper note that he dealt with a relatively small number of cases and he offered no evidence to link leukemia with fallout. But neither could anyone offer any acceptable reasons for the spike in leukemia during the period studied. Said Lyon, "The presumption is that the increase in leukemia is due to atom-bomb tests. While the evidence is circumstantial, we can't find anything else to explain the finding."

The number of leukemia cases for the cohort at Smokey was substantially greater than the predicted incidence for such a sampling of the population. But as Caldwell is quick to note, the question, as in Niles, Illinois, is whether Smokey was a chance event."

For ex-paratrooper Paul Cooper, the results were academic. He died within a month of the subcommittee hearing, more than a year before Caldwell completed his investigations. The other eight leukemia patients, including Donald Coe, were also dead. Coe had been awarded a VA pension on the grounds not of Smokey but that he had been present at a number of tests and had exhibited some signs of illness while still in service. No veteran received a pension purely for having been a witness at an A-bomb test and subsequently, more than eighteen months after receiving an honorable discharge, sickening with a disease that might possibly be connected with radiation exposure. Caldwell's study offered no support for Russell Jack Dann's contention that his troubles were due to Smokey.

Although an encyclopedic range of ailments as a result of exposures at A-bomb tests had been mentioned by veterans of the nuclear experiments, Caldwell could only see epidemic increases in leukemia and skin cancers (which does not eliminate the possibility that an individual with a high susceptibility to some disorder might not have been affected by the radiation).

He did not attempt to determine whether birth defects might have been a consequence of presence at an A-bomb test. "Exposure of a living egg or an embryo does produce mutations. We know that. But that isn't what happened at Smokey. [Pregnant women did not participate in the nuclear tests.] The Japanese cannot find any genetic effects in enzymes and proteins of people who lived through Hiroshima or Nagasaki. They have found some chromosome aberrations, but then chemicals, drugs, spinach, coffee, and radiation can all be associated with chromosome variations. The Japanese cannot find any difference in the offspring of people who were conceived and born by parents who had been irradiated at the two cities." That is, he hastens to add, based on a very small sample; even in Japan it is not that common to find many children with both parents as survivors of the bomb, or who were conceived after both of their parents went through Hiroshima or Nagasaki. There were some microcephalic children; these were in utero at the time of the explosions.

In survivors of the nuclear holocausts, the Japanese found no epidemic increase in blood pressure. They did see higher rates of breast and thyroid cancer as well as leukemia.

The experience at Hiroshima and Nagasaki established beyond doubt that high levels of radiation (about 100 rem at a single shot) lead to serious increases in the sickness rate. None of the hundreds of thousands of U. S. observers at tests received anything near that level. But the question being debated, and of which Smokey has become part of the argument, is what is the long-term effect of low-level radiation, exposure to only 1 to 5 rads.

There is very little evidence upon which to make a judgment. Exposure to radiation of this type is perhaps 35 years old; and many of the men absorbed their ionizing particles and rays as little as 20 to 25 years ago, when they were quite young. Their defects may surface only when they reach their late 50s and 60s.

The Japanese statistics are helpful but not conclusive. Caldwell notes that there was a much higher association of human damage with the Hiroshima detonation than with Nagasaki. He attributes this to the difference in A-bombs. At Hiroshima, the device released many more neutrons. These are the deadliest of the atom bomb's products. Unfortunately, even the makers of the bomb are uncertain of the neutron effects at Hiroshima.

The debate on low-level radiation pits two diametrically opposed points of view. One side insists that there is a threshold level for radiation; that humans tolerate radiation up to that threshold. The trick has been to determine what is that limit. Not surprisingly, those who most strongly advocate the uses of nuclear energy believe in the threshold theory and the only question within that group is where to set the threshold, currently at 5 rem per year for an adult. Since radiation exposure is cumulative, however, some of the threshold school also believe in an upper limit for the duration of one's life.

Challenging this theory are those who insist that radiation risk is linear; it increases almost from zero. One of the more articulate advocates, Dr. Karl Morgan, says the risk begins with only .8 rad exposure. At the House subcommittee hearing, Morgan said, ". . . an overwhelming amount of data have been accumulated that show there is no safe level of exposure and no dose of radiation [so small] that the risk of it causing a malignancy is zero.

Caldwell is unwilling to declare his investigation as grist for either camp. "Smokey is a study of a group of men at one place at one time, not a study of low-dosage radiation. But at least for me the findings raise some important questions. Is it possible that low-level radiation does over a long period of time cause leukemia, unlike the much quicker development of the disease after Hiroshima, where the exposures initially were much higher?"

He seems bemused by the turmoil around Smokey. "Looking back at Smokey, it all started out so innocuously. Someone said, 'Let's give that project to Glyn,' and so I started and the first thing I heard was you can't do this or that, there's no data. And then when we accumulated all the information, the problem became trying to write a finish to the project.

"From March of '76 until the end of '79 it was a real hassle. I felt I was dealing with a small group of people involved in a radiation accident. Part of the fascination is in finding out whether the way you think an investigation will go pans out. This one didn't meet that notion. I was relieved that we didn't find a disaster. I was annoyed in the sense that we didn't do a good study; the information was acquired by cussed persistence, not by dint of scientific design. It was time-consuming but not going to be a major help for other people. I thought there might be new data, social relief for people, some major new scientific contribution. But we couldn't give a good answer to the question of how big a radiation dose does damage. I am pleased that I have done a difficult piece of work. I have learned more about radiation as a virologist and internist."

What does it all mean? "We looked," says Campbell. "It needs a better look. It may solve a whole series of public perceptions by offering some facts, but I don't think it's going to change people's minds.

"When we look at radiation exposure we have to look at a lot of things. There is considerable concern that therapies involving radiation convert to leukemia. Low dosage may be necessary to survive for five years but it may cause something else. The research into low-dosage radiation is extremely important because of the question of cost benefits. Is the chemotherapy or radiotherapy going to produce something worse than the disease? A barium enema [a procedure to detect stomach ulcers and other digestive disorders] means 5 rems exposure. How do you decide whether it's worth doing?"

Although it consumed four years and at the end Caldwell remains uncertain whether he saw horses or zebras, he continues to be enthusiastic. "I'm crazy about my job; it's always different. We're now moving in on evaluations of toxic-waste dumps."

Caldwell is a pioneer in a new frontier of medicine, one that seeks to explore the long-term effects of environment, whether natural or man-made, upon human health. Poisonous refuse is an even younger concern than nuclear-bomb radiation. Smokey offers a preliminary model for looking at the long-term effects of noxious chemicals, a way to separate the horses from the zebras. Caldwell himself is chary of any predictions on what will be found. "We know what radiation may do; with many of these chemicals we don't even know what to look for." But he intends to keep looking, as long as he hears the sound of hoofbeats. Indeed, the CDC has now been assigned the task of investigating the possible effects of the defoliant, Agent Orange, upon U.S. troops who served in Vietnam, and Caldwell will not be surprised if he is tapped for some part of the study.

CHAPTER
6

TSS

A YOUNG MOTHER named Linda Riccardi noticed one day that her two-year-old son was slightly feverish and had broken out in a rash. The family pediatrician prescribed an antibiotic, and the boy recovered. But two days later Linda Riccardi herself developed a headache and slight fever. Her doctor assumed she had contracted her son's infection. An antibiotic appeared to clear the infection. But several days later Mrs. Riccardi suffered a relapse. Her temperature shot up. She shivered from chills. Nausea and stomach cramps were followed by severe diarrhea.

"I could hardly get out of bed," says Mrs. Riccardi. "I called the doctor and told him, but he was not able to see me until the next day." She felt so weak that two people had to assist her to visit the physician. The doctor drew blood for a lab test and sent his patient home.

On the following day the doctor's nurse telephoned and instructed Mrs. Riccardi to see a surgeon. The sick woman felt confused. Hardly able to think and talk coherently, she managed to arrange an appointment with the surgeon at the local hospital's emergency room. When she arrived, in her words, she was "cramped over in pain, had a high fever, was vomiting bile, and had continuous diarrhea. I was pale and drawn. My eyes were sunken and had dark rings."

The surgeon found her white cell count five to ten times above normal, a sign of a severe infection. An exploratory abdominal operation was inconclusive. "I thought I was going to die," Mrs. Riccardi recalls. "I woke up in intensive care after surgery with a tube down my nose and stomach and I had a heart catheter."

Mrs. Riccardi was suffering from the now famous toxic shock syndrome (TSS), a condition for which millions of American women suddenly were found at risk. A number of victims died while others were left with a lifetime disability. The problem involved a $500 million business, spotlighted the question of governmental responsibility for protection of consumers, and to this day remains a threat.

It all began with a puzzle stumping Dr. Joan Chesney, a pediatric infectious disease expert in Madison, Wisconsin. Dr. Chesney was disturbed by the symptoms of three female patients, 15, 18, and 25 years of age, in West Madison. They had all run temperatures of 102°F. or higher, broken out in a diffuse body rash, and suffered a significant drop in blood pressure. In varying degrees, the patients complained of stomach distress—vomiting or diarrhea—and muscular aches. Accompanying the fever peaks were episodes of delirium. One of the trio had lapsed into kidney failure and required the use of a dialysis machine to perform the functions normally rendered by the kidneys. Finally, even as all three began to show signs of recovery, skin peeled away from the palms of their hands and the soles of their feet.

About the same time, Dr. Gerald Shrock, a Minneapolis physician, was also deeply mystified by his experience with a patient. The 20-year-old woman had come down with a fever, gastrointestinal pains, and a rash. She did not respond to treatment and died within a few days. Immediately, Shrock notified Dr. Michael T. Osterholm, chief of acute-disease epidemiology in the Minnestota State Department of Health.

"Even as we were discussing this case," recalls Osterholm, "Shrock reported that he had a second young woman with the same symptoms." Checking other local doctors, Osterholm learned of several more physicians wrestling with the same syndrome. One more death had been reported.

The Minnesota State Health Department's chief epidemiologist, Dr. Andrew Dean, telephoned his opposite number in Wisconsin, Dr. Jeffrey Davis. Both had served in the EIS, Davis having arrived in Atlanta one year earlier than Dean.

The latter took notes on their conversation, which was as follows: "Hi, Jeff, this is Andy Dean. Say, we've had two deaths here in young people, and I wanted to ask—"

"Wait. I'll bet they're in young women with an erythromatous rash and fever."

"How did you know?"

"We've had five cases over here since September. It's called toxic shock syndrome. Look at Todd's article in the *Lancet* for November 1978."

"We've had four cases in Minnesota. Do you know of any others?"

"I think there is one in Oklahoma."

"We'd better call the CDC and see if they know of any others," concluded Dean.

That afternoon Dean called Atlanta. However, the CDC watchman who answered the telephone resisted putting Dean in touch with a professional from the Special Pathogens Branch. "I finally told him," says Dean, "that we had a problem with Legionnaires' disease."

At the CDC, David Fraser (who had led the investigation into Legionnaires' disease; see Chapter 2) nominated Kathryn Shands to oversee TSS. "I was the only EIS officer in the unit who had more than a year left to serve, and would be able to follow it through," explains Shands, a handsome, willowy young woman in her early 30s.

As an adolescent Kathy Shands dreamed of following in the footsteps of her physician father. "He discouraged me, telling me that it was too rough a road for a woman, saying I'd have to give up too much of life and femininity for a medical career. As a teenager I accepted what he said.

"I majored in English and psychology as an undergraduate at Cornell, and when I graduated took a job at Massachusetts General Hospital in news and publications. It didn't satisfy me, and I became involved with the language clinic. I was supposed to work with dyslexia and wound up teaching reading to failing kids.

"I went out to California and when I couldn't find a job in the field of dyslexia, went to work for the welfare department. Then I spent a year assisting a psychologist.

"The writing on the wall became clear to me during these years. I was not going to be satisfied until I became a doctor. I spent two years taking courses that would make me eligible for medical school and was accepted at Boston University

Medical School." She specialized in pediatrics and went on to a fellowship in pediatric infections.

"During a course in community medicine while at Boston University," says Shands, "I discovered the story of John Snow and cholera. I was fascinated, but I thought to myself, it's too bad that kind of work can't be done in this day and age."

She responded with skepticism to the suggestion that she try to follow Snow's path by means of the CDC. "I said I don't want a lab job, but a teacher explained it's not lab work." And so Shands became an EIS officer in the summer of 1979.

Shands started her investigation by studying the paper on toxic shock syndrome written by Dr. James Todd, a Colorado physician. For Todd, the index case, the one central to the description of TSS, was that of a 15-year-old girl who had entered Denver's Children's Hospital with a fever of 105.62°F. She was "confused," "aggressive," and in a state of shock. Her systolic blood pressure fell to 66. She went through episodes of vomiting and diarrhea and a red rash—a diffuse erythroderma—covered her entire body. She received a battery of therapies, intravenous fluids, antibiotics, steroid drugs, digitalis, heparin, oxygen—altogether a heroic effort was made on her behalf. On the third day of her hospitalization, skin peeled from her feet and abdomen, but she had begun to recover. After a week in the hospital she was discharged, minus two toes on her left foot, which had been amputated after the onset of gangrene.

Todd, a pediatrician, and some associates had seen this peculiar medical problem in three boys and three more girls between the ages of 8 and 17. One youngster had died. Todd noted that all his charges had "fine desquamation"—peeling of skin from the palms and soles during convalescence. The symptoms common to all included persistent lowering of blood pressure, the rash, and elevated temperatures, along with gastrointestinal troubles and some mental confusion.

Laboratory workups, which included help from the CDC, had ruled out fungus infections, Rocky Mountain spotted fever, and streptococcal bacteria. What did show in five of the kids was the presence of a common bacterium, *Staphylococcus aureus*, or staph aureus, which is known to produce on occasion a toxic byproduct. Todd wrote up his findings for the British medical journal, the *Lancet*, and concluded, ". . . the acute illness which we have described and called toxic shock syndrome seems to affect older children."

Nothing more was heard on the subject, but one of the people who had read Todd's paper was Jeff Davis, who had long puzzled over a patient he had seen while a pediatric resident at the Duke University Medical School and whose symptoms matched those described by the Colorado doctor. When Joan Chesney reported her experiences, Davis immediately tied her description with Todd's toxic shock syndrome, which quickly assumed the abbreviation TSS in medical literature.

The CDC's effort at this point was low-keyed. Kathy Shands frequently chatted about the matter with a jogging partner who had the office across the hall from her, Dr. Bruce Dan, whose EIS assignment was the CDC's Hospital Infections Branch. "When I first came to the CDC in July of 1979," says the bearded Dan, "I met this tall woman in the EIS class. In the course of conversation I said I was going to run in the Boston Marathon. She said she'd meet me at the 24-mile mark with a beer and a kiss. I forgot about it, but she was there with both. Kathy Shands has been my best friend ever since."

They make a somewhat disparate pair. Shands is more cautious and less impulsive than Dan, whose candor is frequently alien to what's considered good form in a government worker or scientist.

Bruce Dan's route to the CDC and the toxic shock syndrome investigation was even more circuitous than that of Kathy Shands. Dan started out as an aeronautical engineer with a Bachelor of Science degree from MIT. He pursued further education in that field as a graduate student at Purdue. "One morning around 6:45 I was on my way to teach a class. It was cold, gray outside. I started to think about my career, what am I doing with my life. I came into the building for my class; it was quiet, the only sound was the whoosh of the ventilating system. I asked myself, Is this how I want to spend my time? What should I do? From out of nowhere, from behind me, came a voice: 'Go to medical school.' Of course, there was nobody there.

"I gave my class an assignment to work out and I rushed

over to the placement office, which was just opening up. 'How do I get into medical school? What's the best one? What subjects do I have to take?' They didn't believe I was serious; finally they accepted that my desire was real. I needed some biology courses. I went to see the instructor; she said I didn't have the prerequisites. I insisted I could do the work. She said okay, if you pass the test. I went home and studied for forty-eight hours, then came back and took the exam. The teacher called me: 'What is this, a joke? You're a graduate student, you got an A.' We became friends. I made up the biology requirements, but it was too late for me to get into medical school that year, so I had to wait." In the interim, Dan worked at Massachusetts General Hospital as an engineer and computer scientist and then was employed by the National Aeronautical and Space Agency in its biotechnology division before entering Vanderbilt University Medical School. During his sojourn in Tennessee, Dan witnessed a CDC investigation into an epidemic of sorts, an antibiotic-resistant infection. Encouraged by an enthusiastic alumnus on the faculty at Vanderbilt, Dan obtained an EIS appointment. By the time he had enlisted in the program, Dan also had been certified in internal medicine and done fellowships in infectious diseases and computer medicine.

After he had been actually detailed to the investigation of TSS, Dan visited a patient in an Atlanta hospital. "It's one thing to hear about a disease on the telephone," says he, "and another to actually see it. I wrote a memo in which I said, 'I've seen a lot of infectious diseases, but I never saw anything like this. It's a whole new phenomenon. There are limited ways a body can react to some stimuli; a rash, fever. But here is a constellation of injuries, a fever of 106° or 107°, unheard of in an adult, a rash, muscle soreness, enzyme changes, kidney, brain, liver, heart, all involved.' I had never seen such an acute result of some toxic substance."

An apparent handful of cases in Minnesota and Wisconsin suggested that TSS was no longer a medical-journal oddity. However, the CDC required solid epidemiological evidence on the actual extent of the problem. But before that could be determined, there had to be agreement on what constituted a case of TSS. By telephone, Shands discussed the available information with Jeff Davis, and then flew to Denver to confer with James Todd and Dr. Neal Halsey, who held a CDC fellowship in pediatric infectious diseases at the University of Colorado Medical Center. They worked out a rather stringent case definition of toxic shock syndrome. It specified four symptoms. There had to be sudden onset of a high fever, almost always about 104°F; vomiting and diarrhea; rapid progression toward low blood pressure (below 90 systolic for adults, which indicates shock); and finally, a sunburn-like rash followed by scalelike peeling on the soles of the feet and palms of the hands.

The condition began with a staphylococcus infection, and the bacterium then produced a toxic substance which damaged the capillaries, causing blood to leak into the tissues, destroying them, and reducing blood pressure. With the case definition set, the task force began to check with other state health departments for their experience with TSS.

Even as Shands and Dan began to accumulate information, preliminary research by Osterholm in Minnesota and Davis in Wisconsin made apparent two significant facts about the current cases of TSS. They were almost entirely confined to young women with onset during their menstrual periods. "It wasn't difficult to make the connection," says Davis. "All of the patients were female, and when you check the records you found that in every instance the person became sick during her menstrual period." Indeed, Linda Riccardi's sudden turn for the worse coincided with the onset of menstruation.

But just as the first phase of the investigation, the case definition and toting up of preliminary numbers, got underway, both Shands and Dan were called for duty elsewhere. Shands went to California for two months to investigate the Wadsworth Hospital Legionnaires' disease. Dan was tapped to serve as chief medical officer at the Fort Chaffee, Arkansas, center for Cuban refugees. "It was a shock to me," says Dan. "I had just finished a course in Spanish, fortunately, but it was bizarre suddenly being put in charge of the health of 20,000 people. I was given the rank of a military major and I had to learn how to salute while dealing with outbreaks of food poisoning, meningitis, Green Berets."

In May, however, the CDC operatives were all back on the case, and with Shands as chief and Dan as her deputy, a task force devoted its full time to it. The task force reported directly to David Fraser, as chief of the Special Pathogens Branch. The CDC went public with the problem through the May 23 issue of the *Morbidity and Mortality Weekly Report* (*MMWR*), which announced that since October 1, 1979, fifty-five cases of TSS had been reported and fifty-two of them were women, almost all of whom said the onset of illness followed the start of the menstrual period. Three-quarters of the patients harbored a staph aureus infection. The case-fatality rate was placed at 10-15 percent, extremely high.

Once again the media descended on the CDC. Kathy Shands met with a reporter from the *Washington Post* who is a physician. The questions were professional, and Shands relaxed. Toward the end of the interview, the writer asked if the whole business wasn't "scary." Shands agreed. She was taken aback to see herself quoted in the lead to the *Post* piece as saying the whole business was "scary." From then on Shands measured her words and avoided any comments that might sensationalize the problem.

The choice of a woman, Shands, to lead the TSS task force originally may have been fortuitous, but she remarks, "Don Berreth [head of the CDC's public information office] thought it was a good idea for a woman to talk to reporters on the subject. There were direct questions. Had I made any change in my tampon habits? I answered that the CDC recommended that women need not change their tampon-using habits. I think that carried some weight."

Even as the preliminary announcements about TSS appeared, Osterholm and Davis had noted another significant aspect of the cases. Not only were the women in their menstrual period but they all appeared to use tampons rather than some other method of coping with the flow of menses. Bruce Dan points out, "When you have a large number of cases which are women that are not the same age and a large percentage get sick during the menstrual period, it's not likely a matter of random chance. You ask yourself what's happening in menstruating women. One possibility is that they're taking medicine for cramps and somehow they got a bad batch of the medicine. But that didn't prove out, and when the women were asked about their habits during menstruation, the correlation with tampons showed up."

Says Shands, "We did a quick telephone case control survey.

We contacted fifty-two women who had had toxic shock syndrome and an equal number of their friends who did not. In addition, the women were questioned about their marital status, contraceptive methods, frequency of sexual intercourse, and the brand of tampon or sanitary napkin used. At the same time we asked the manufacturers of products for absorbing menstrual flow how many women used tampons. It came to 70 percent. We also requested data on the products, the chemical components, the absorbency, and their marketing practices."

The tabulated responses showed clearly that tampons and menstruation were closely connected with TSS. Linda Riccardi routinely used tampons during her periods.

Shands and Dan briefed the upper echelons of the CDC. Arrangements were made to inform both the tampon manufacturers and the Food and Drug Administration, the federal agency with responsibility for monitoring products such as tampons.

The major makers of tampons agreed to meet with the toxic shock syndrome task force in Atlanta on June 24 to discuss the CDC's findings and to exchange further information. While awaiting these sessions, Shands, Dan, and associates drafted a second report for the *MMWR*.

The initial meetings were pleasant and without any adversarial quality. The manufacturers received copies of the draft of the *MMWR* report. "We told them we'd listen to what they had to say, and we made some changes in a few words at their request," says Shands. "They were sensitive about the marketing aspects of the problem. But the facts were not altered in the report."

The latest *MMWR*, summarizing the new studies, noted that 42 percent of the Wisconsin patients experienced at least one recurrence of TSS. There were no significant differences or trends uncovered in the contraceptive methods, the number of sexual partners, whether sexual intercourse occurred during menstruation, history of herpes infections, previous vaginal infections, or uses of douches or sprays during menstruation.

The report noted that while TSS was associated with tampon use during menstruation, particularly continual use, the role played by the tampon was still a mystery. Furthermore, the incidence of TSS appeared to be very low; Wisconsin was reporting about three cases per 100,000 menstruating women.

The *MMWR* specifically stated that no particular brand of tampon was associated with a high risk of TSS but that tampons might favor the growth of bacteria or the absorption of the toxin produced by staph aureus. The report saw no great risk for the vast majority of women using tampons but recommended that women who had suffered TSS should "probably not" use tampons for several menstrual cycles after their illness or until they were certain that any staph aureus infec-infection in the vagina had been eradicated.

By midsummer, 171 confirmed cases of TSS had been reported to the CDC, with twelve deaths. Shands, Dan, and two associates, Dr. George Schmid and Dr. Wally Schlech, over the weekend of September 5-8 questioned fifty women who had come down with TSS during July and August. Their pattern of tampon use was compared with that of 150 healthy women, and something that had been missed in the earlier surveys appeared: An extremely high percentage of those with toxic shock syndrome used a particular tampon, the RELY brand made by Procter & Gamble. Plans were made to publish the results in the *MMWR* of September 19.

Aware now of the economic stakes, the task force met with superiors, including Dr. John Bennett, director of the Bacterial Diseases Division of the Bureau of Epidemiology, and Dr. Phillip S. Brachman, director of the Bureau of Epidemiology. Brachman departed the next day to advise Surgeon General Julius Richmond on the findings. The TSS task force also conferred with CDC director Dr. William Foege, and he informed the Food and Drug Administration. Officials from that agency flew to Atlanta to discuss the matter. By September 15, Shands, Foege, Dan, and Schmid were all in the nation's capital to explain the situation to Health and Human Services Secretary Patricia Harris, Surgeon General Richmond, and FDR Commissioner Dr. Jere Goyan.

TSS became a highly charged matter. On the surface this was a rather rare ailment; the official statistics now put the incidence at six cases per 100,000 menstruating women in the United States (it was less than one per 100,000 for women who did not use tampons). But on the other hand, 50 million women who used tampons were potentially at risk. Short of giving up a convenient product there appeared no way of ensuring protection for a woman of childbearing age. And because so many women and a common commercial item were involved the economic stakes were enormous.

Linkage of tampons with the devastation wrought by TSS would inevitably cut deeply into the $500 million market for the product. Manufacturers would probably be hit with multi-million-dollar lawsuits from women who developed the illness —some of whom were permanently injured—or from the survivors of those wives and mothers who died of TSS. The Federal Trade Commission would have to decide whether to declare a single brand or all tampons dangerous, whether to require that one or all be withdrawn from sale, or whether to insist that every package, as with cigarettes, carry a warning that the product might be injurious to health.

The CDC had now entered a highly sensitive area. It is not empowered to control the sale or distribution of a product such as a tampon. That was the responsibility of the FDA. On the other hand, findings by the CDC can cause regulatory agencies to issue bans on items and move Congress to pass legislation restricting the manufacture of products.

Tampons had been classified by the FDA as medical devices in 1976, and as such they were regarded as a Class II product. Items in this category are those in which enough is believed known about the materials and the manufacturing process to allow performance standards to be written. But five years after the legislation authorizing these standards, the FDA still has none. Along with tampons, Class II includes hearing aids, incubators, and devices to monitor pregnancies.

For all tampons, therefore, the regulation by the government consists of having a record of the materials employed in the product. That is not to say that the manufacturers did not extensively test their merchandise. For RELY there was a long period of design and experimentation. It included even the insertion of tiny facsimiles of RELY in rabbits. (Unfortunately, TSS cannot be replicated in animals.) There were some complaints initially about problems with RELY—none having to do with TSS—and the company over the years made a number of changes in both materials and design as the product went national.

The comings and goings, the contacting of the topmost federal officials, demonstrates an awareness of the sensitivity of the subject and the determination of CDC chiefs both to protect the CDC and to leave no opportunity for those with a financial interest to cry foul.

Representatives of the various manufacturers of tampons came to Washington to confer there with Shands and Dan, among others. "We met individually with Procter & Gamble," recalls Shands, "and then with all of the manufacturers. We gave P&G a summary of our data. They happened to have already scheduled a meeting of their scientific advisory board and it was agreed that the company could have a week to respond. But they also wanted to meet immediately with Foege—that night, in fact." The reason for the haste was obvious; publication of the *MMWR* laying out the case against RELY was only three days off.

"They offered to fly us down to Atlanta in their plane," remembers Dan. "We called Foege and he said, 'No way.' We went by commercial airplane and they traveled separately in their company plane."

At 7:00 a.m. on the morning of September 17, the representatives of P&G along with the members of the TSS task force sat down with Foege. Shands remembers that the major thrust of the discussion was a plea to delay the publication of the *MMWR*. P&G asked that the data be submitted to an independent research group for review before publication. Foege politely listened and then said the matter was too important to postpone. From Atlanta, the P&G group flew back to Washington for one last try: an appeal to Patricia Harris, who in her capacity as head of HEW could have overruled Foege. She declined. They sought out Congressmen from Ohio (headquarters of P&G are in Cincinnati), but no help came from that quarter. As a courtesy, the CDC turned over to P&G copies of its computer runs, all of the data upon which the indictment of RELY was based.

On September 19, as planned, the third *MMWR* report on TSS appeared. It summarized the previous publications and brought the figures up to date: 299 cases of TSS reported, 285 in women, with twenty-five deaths, an 8.4 percent rate. Approximately 95 percent of TSS in women occurred during a menstrual period.

The report showed that 71 percent of the women with TSS used the RELY brand. Playtex tampons were involved in 19 percent of the TSS cases. Tampax tampons were involved in 5 percent, and two other brands, Kotex and QB, accounted for 2 percent each. Mrs. Riccardi's brand had been Tampax.

Predictably, some of the public, particularly victims, reacted strongly to the disclosures. Cynthia Bendoraitis of Oak Lawn, Illinois, who spent five days in Christ Hospital's intensive-care ward before recovering from TSS, said, "When they come out with a tampon, doesn't the government have to inspect it or something? Or can they just put things on the market?" Under the prevailing policies of the FDA, companies could.

Linda Imboden of Redding, California, who lost her waist-length hair and lost sensation in her fingertips and toes because of gangrene and whose hands were deformed into curvelike claws after a bout with TSS, sued P&G for $5 million.

On Monday, September 22, the CDC task force was again in Washington to discuss with the FDA the next step. Midway through the discussions, they were interrupted by a report taken from the wire services which said that Procter & Gamble had announced it would withdraw RELY tampons from the market. The company's scientific advisory group, which had convened over the weekend, had looked over the CDC data and, while they had some minor quibbles, felt the case was too strong to be fought.

It is Shand's memory of the experience that the officials of P&G always "behaved like gentlemen, quite reasonable, except they were tough on legal material. They had a lot of skepticism about our findings, plenty of criticism, but it was in terms of the language we used rather than the data."

Bruce Dan does not see the manufacturers as quite so benign. "At first they said what we had was 'wonderful stuff, but we haven't had time to go over it.' But when it became clear that they would have to respond to the FDA in a week and we meant to go ahead with publication, things got rough. 'What if you're wrong?' they said. 'We're a responsible company. It involves thousands of workers.' We answered, 'What if you're wrong? Women have died.' All they wanted to talk about was possible litigation."

Dan also found the FDA reluctant to apply pressure. "The FDA likes to avoid problems. It isn't like the CDC, where you deal with unknowns and stresses, where you have people

coming down sick with things you don't understand and where
people die around you. The FDA is just a bureaucracy, a
regulatory agency that likes its ducks in order. This was a
very uncertain situation, not to their liking, but we zapped it.
We twisted their arms, telling them we were going to publish,
and only then would they move."

The CDC team also found itself in the politics of medical
publishing. A treatise was submitted to the *New England
Journal of Medicine*. About the same time, Jeff Davis independently submitted his own paper on the subject. Shands,
Dan, and associates claim the journal said it could not publish
two items on this subject and asked that the material be combined. The CDC team refused to accede to the request; the
journal, after six weeks, returned the CDC proposal.

When the *MMWR* appeared with the material on RELY
and TSS, Arnold Relman, editor of the *New England Journal
of Medicine*, asked the CDC people to resubmit their paper.
It was published in the December 1980 issue of the journal.
Bruce Dan remarks, "It was a sorry state when for six months
women had to bring newspaper articles to their doctors about
toxic shock because a medical journal rejected publication of
the paper." A scornful Dan notes, "Not a single word was
changed from what we submitted originally to what was
finally published. Indeed, the paper which was written in July
did not mention differences in tampon brands. It was only
because of the material in the *MMWR* on RELY that they
were forced to take our piece."

While Dan's conclusion might be challenged by the editors
of the *New England Journal of Medicine*, the delayed publication, according to Kathy Shands, introduced a new note of
confusion. "Coming out *after* the *MMWR* on RELY, the
journal piece caused some people to think that this was new
information and that RELY had been exonerated."

Conceivably, the failure of a paper on TSS to appear
promptly in a medical journal hindered a rapid diagnosis of
Linda Riccardi's sickness. The onset of her toxic shock occurred in October, almost four months after the first *MMWR*
but two months before there was a discussion in a professional
magazine that might have informed her doctor. When her
exploratory surgery was inconclusive, her physicians telephoned the CDC to describe the symptoms and determine if

these fitted the disease being publicized by the popular media. Only then was she started on a course of anti-staph-aureus drugs and intravenous fluids that enabled her to survive.

Although RELY is now off the market and an impartial organization, the Institute of Medicine from the National Academy of Sciences, agreed with the CDC's conclusions about the relative involvement of tampons, neither the problems of TSS nor the question of RELY's involvement have vanished.

"We could not confirm in the laboratory what we knew from our epidemiological study, but TSS was not exclusively limited to women using RELY. We took whole tampons as well as components of them," explains Shands, "soaked them in blood and inoculated them with staph aureus. But we couldn't see any difference between one tampon and another in the lab.

"Even when RELY was named as a potential cause," recalls Shands, "we were getting calls from people who insisted that it was the best tampon ever made. We also heard from those who said our finding about RELY was the best thing the CDC has ever done. There were maybe eighty to a hundred calls a day, fifty letters a day, mostly from women who thought they had toxic shock, but there were also physicians who had some ideas, and then there were all of the reporters.

"We knew we're not getting all the cases," says Shands. "We sacrificed numbers for more exact diagnoses. There were people who wanted an even stricter definition of TSS and there were those who wanted a more liberal one. We probably ruled out some women with TSS but we wanted to be certain we eliminated any other illnesses that might have confused the investigation. Ours was strictly an epidemiological definition. It could help us see trends and set up control cases, find risk factors."

Art Reingold, a University of Chicago Medical School graduate, had become a member of the task force almost immediately after he joined the EIS. "I like my job," said Reingold at the time. "I like it because it's the closest I can get to cheap sleazy detective work. This way I can make a living and not get shot. I've always wanted to be a detective, and this comes pretty close."

Reingold noted, "All states have certain diseases physicians are required to report. In general, the more common the disease, the less it is reported. Measles is way underreported. Salmonella is supposed to be reported; the percent reported is small. There are also some diseases that get very careful reporting, like polio, botulism, of course, because the physician has to obtain the antitoxin, rabies, diphtheria. TSS is not legally reportable. We hear about cases but there's no obligation upon a doctor. Some of the physicians have offered information because they've heard about TSS in the press and because it's interesting. But as time has passed, the cases are no longer something new, they're not as interesting, they know how to treat it, and it is now routine. They don't call us. A guy or gal will still get excited when he or she sees his first case. You also get patients who want to be diagnosed as toxic shock syndrome because they want to sue somebody and they want the state health officials to testify on their behalf."

There is now full agreement that a staph infection is already present in the vagina at the time a woman uses a tampon. "A tampon helps set up a site for the infection to thrive," says Shands. "One theory on how staph aureus gets into the bloodstream is that the tampon causes slight, even microscopic tears in the lining of the vagina, permitting the infection to enter the bloodstream.

"We haven't been able to determine this through clinical examination," she adds. "When a woman comes into the emergency room in toxic shock, nobody wants to put her up in stirrups and have a gynecologist with a coposcope [an instrument for viewing the vagina] looking at her vagina for thirty minutes to find any microabscesses or microlacerations."

The connection of superabsorbent tampons with TSS suggested to some that the efficiency of the product was responsible. In this theory the tampon absorbed not only the menstrual blood but also the fluids that lubricate the membranes of the vagina. As a result the tissue became dry and easily ulcerated, opening up an avenue for staph infection to flourish.

Meanwhile, the discussion over the extent of TSS continues. As many as 13 percent of the total reported cases have not involved menstruating women. TSS has been found in postsurgical patients, in victims of burns, in women immediately after childbirth, and even in people with minor boils or abscesses.

The feeling is that like legionella, toxic shock syndrome has been around for a considerable period of time. As early as 1927, someone described "staphylococcal scarlet fever," which most likely was TSS. "In going over medical records," says Reingold, "we see most cases that were probably TSS had been labeled as adult Kawasaki disease of unknown origins. Kawasaki is a sickness common in Japan, usually in children, and it has similar symptoms. Sometimes we think the disease was diagnosed as scarlet fever, Rocky Mountain spotted fever, and leptospirosis."

Some scientists feel the sudden appearance of TSS and its subsequent waning has less to do with reporting and diagnosis than with the elusive nature of the staphylococcus beast, which ebbs and flows with different strains. Another question concerns the selectivity of the disease. Another hypothesis is that the victims—mostly younger women—had less previous exposure to staph infections and fewer antibodies. They were also primarily white, from families with incomes in the $15,000 to $25,000 range. Perhaps these women came from homes with better than average sanitary conditions; they avoided early exposure to staph infections and developed no resistance to them. Certainly Linda Riccardi fits this theory.

"What we need," said Shands, "is a simple diagnostic test. There have been some promising leads on discovering the toxin, but nothing concrete yet. If we knew the toxin we could draw a blood sample and a urine sample to find it. Even when TSS is properly diagnosed, the physician still finds himself in difficult straits. Once the poison is in the bloodstream there is no antitoxin to counteract it, only supportive therapy until the patient's own system disposes of the noxious element. Appropriate antibiotics for a staph infection can halt the manufacture of the toxin or at least prevent reinfection."

For all of the pressure-cooker atmosphere—Kathy Shands shoving a tampon across the desk to HEW Secretary Harris by way of explaining its role, appearances on network programs such as *The Today Show*, the *MacNeil-Lehrer Report*, and *Good Morning America*, the crash surveys over weekends, the confrontations with high-powered lawyers and executives from major U.S. companies, the sense of being at the center of the action—task-force members did not escape the touch of human suffering. "A woman died of toxic shock," recalls Reingold. "She had just gotten married. She became ill on her honeymoon and died. Her husband called us. 'I really want to come down and talk to someone,' he said. He wanted to find out what was going on with the investigation and whether he could help. I told him I could tell him over the telephone, but if he had the need to talk to someone I would see him. He came. I spent three hours with him. I showed him around. I talked to him about research. He had the need to feel that something was being done. So I think his coming and talking to someone was helpful to him."

It fell to Shands to speak to the family of one of the earliest cases. "A young woman had died. I got calls from her father, her mother, and her husband, all of whom wanted to give me whatever information they could." And throughout the investigation the task-force members, although removed from the ordinary day-to-day contact of the practice of medicine, made it their business to offer a sympathetic ear and a counseling voice to worried women who called or wrote about their fears.

While Linda Riccardi was still in bed recuperating from her attack of TSS, she began to research the disease. "At that time I did a lot of thinking and reading. I was determined to find out why I got sick and how." When she had recovered completely she added one more activity to her career as a businesswoman, mother, and wife—she became a speaker on the subject of TSS before local civic groups.

The original task force assigned to TSS broke up eighteen months after the start of the investigation. The paper submitted by the group and published in the *New England Journal of Medicine* won the CDC's 1981 Alexander D. Langmuir Prize Manuscript award.

Kathy Shands found separation from the CDC difficult. When she completed her term as an EIS officer she received a fellowship in infectious diseases in Boston. But an administrative post with the CDC opened up, and she accepted it. After six months, however, Shands said, "I realize I'm not cut out for this kind of work. It's more fun to be an EIS officer. The problem is that it is only a two-year job and there's nothing like it. When you come to the CDC you hear stories about investigations and you say, 'Wow, that's the kind of thing that can happen to me.' But you don't really expect it, yet it happened to me." Shands has decided to pursue a career in child psychiatry.

When his EIS term ended, Bruce Dan left the CDC, but he has stayed in Atlanta. Dan's eyes take on a glow when he talks of his two years in the EIS. "Most EIS officers are people who haven't decided on clear goals. They're restless, they tend to be unmarried. In the EIS you parachute in, maybe you're in charge of the health of hundreds, thousands of people. You're in the trenches. Most places you have a notion that's off the wall and they'll tell you, 'Don't waste your time.' At the CDC they would say, 'Why not look into that?' I could do EIS for twenty years. There's nothing like it."

7

Something Did Not Go
Well with Coke

THE FIRST PATIENT to arrive at the Craven County Hospital in New Bern, North Carolina, was David Keller (pseudonym), a 19-year-old construction worker. When he was admitted on July 9, 1979, Keller was thought to be a flu victim. He had experienced nausea, vomiting, and a general malaise, and his condition seemed to be worsening. Within the next few days three more men between the ages of 18 and 22 were in the same hospital, their symptoms similar to those of David Keller, but no one was talking about flu anymore. Tests from specimens on Keller and the others sent to a nearby lab had revealed definite traces of hepatitis. The appearance of that many cases of the disease was alarming enough, but even more sinister was the severity of the infections. All four patients were in desperate shape.

Attached to the Craven County Hospital was Bobbie Golec, a nurse assigned by the state health department to follow up on any communicable diseases in the county. "The local doctors don't ordinarily stock gamma globulin," explains Nurse Golec, "and when the diagnosis of the first young man came back as hepatitis, the physician referred the family to me at the hospital for a gamma globulin injection as protection. When a second family was referred to me I realized we might have something out of the ordinary on hand. The first two boys were friends, but the third patient did not know the other two. That definitely suggested the possibility of an epidemic. I naturally notified Dr. Barefoot at the county health department."

After hearing the details of the situation, Dr. Verna Barefoot, the Craven County officer, did not hesitate. "I called the CDC on a Saturday evening. It was the first time I ever had to ask for their help. My call to Atlanta," recalls Dr. Barefoot, "was relayed to Phoenix, where I spoke to Dr. Donald Francis. I told him that we had four young people critically ill with hepatitis B."

"It was 10:00 p.m. our time and I was at home," recalls Francis, indicating the concern felt by Dr. Barefoot back in North Carolina, where it was midnight. "What struck me immediately," says Francis, "was that they had four cases of what we call fulminant hepatitis, which is life-threatening. Ordinarily Type B is fatal in about 1 percent of the cases. Since it was July, the CDC was in the midst of training a new set of EIS officers. We did not actually have anyone in Phoenix to send to New Bern. We located the nearest person, Dr. Carl Armstrong, attached to the Virginia Health Department, and he was on the scene the next day. I arrived the following night."

Hepatitis, from the Greek word for "liver," *hepatos*, is a viral disease that attacks the liver and manifests itself in three strains. Infectious hepatitis, Type A, is a common communicable version. It spreads through fecal contamination of food —shellfish, milk, fruit, water—and of clothing, toys, and eating utensils. Frequently mild, Type A may even be free of the yellow tinge of jaundice—in medical terms, "icterus"—usually associated with hepatitis.

Type B, known as serum hepatitis, shows the same symptoms as its kin but is often more severe in its attack. About 10 percent of those who come down with Type B become chronic carriers of the virus in their blood. As a consequence, sharing of personal-hygiene items like toothbrushes and razors can transmit Type B. The disease is also passed through contaminated hypodermic needles by drug users, needles for tattoos, and ear-piercing instruments. Type B can survive in semen, making some homosexuals and prostitutes with their extensive sexual activity at high risk for the disease. Until screening methods improved, blood transfusions were a common source of Type B; now only some technicians (in spite of gloves, sterile gowns, and masks) and people who use dialysis machines (the artificial kidney) are at much risk of infection while handling blood. There is a third and lesser version called Non-A and Non-B. It was discovered when donor blood that had successfully cleared screening for Type B nevertheless produced hepatitis in recipients.

All types of hepatitis are clearly recognizable through specific laboratory tests. Craven County Hospital did not have the facilities for such tests; several days were lost because of the need to send the specimens outside the area for examination. There is no drug or surgical treatment for hepatitis. The cure is a matter of rest and supportive therapy while waiting for the body to overcome the enemy. Gamma globulin injections provide short-term immunity against Type A. But in 1979 there was no vaccine for Type B, and so there was nothing the Craven County Health Department could do to protect local people. They could only warn the community of the ways in which Type B spreads. (In 1982, a vaccine was developed for Type B.)

The CDC's involvement with hepatitis began in the late 1950s when the disease first achieved recognition as a public health problem. Among the very first CDC investigations was that of a new EIS officer, Dr. Bruce H. Dull. He was dispatched to New Jersey in 1961 to track down the source of a Type A outbreak. From the patients, Bruce Dull learned they all had one thing in common: Their physician, who had given them injections during the two-to-eight-week period before they became ill. Interrogating the physician, Dull discovered that he was so busy he frequently did not pause to sterilize equipment between patients. When Dull suggested as tactfully as he could that the doctor possibly was spreading hepatitis, the accused man strenuously protested. Dull had no choice but to present his evidence to the local medical society. It was unprecedented, but Dull's documentation convinced the other professionals. A significant result was the widespread publication of the probability of disease through contaminated needles, even when in the hands of a doctor.

Another landmark investigation into hepatitis followed an epidemic in Pascagoula, Mississippi. EIS officer Dr. James O. Mason was sent by the CDC to look into the affair after a U.S. Navy medical officer became concerned over the number of cases among workers at the Pascagoula shipyard that produced nuclear-powered naval vessels. His worry was that it might spread to critical personnel and their dependents.

Hepatitis was not a reportable disease, and Mason, while he knew of thirteen people hospitalized, was concerned about the extent of the epidemic. Unable to find anyone with figures for the area, he plunked himself down in the doctor's lounge of the Pascagoula Hospital. As physicians halted for a coffee break, Mason interviewed them about their experiences with hepatitis. He not only obtained the names of seventy patients but by the end of the day had narrowed down the source of the disease to raw oysters that came from a particular oyster-man harvesting the shellfish from a site hard by the end of a sewer line. With seafood markets in Mobile, Alabama, selling some of the catch from Pascagoula, the hepatitis epidemic had spread to the neighboring state. Through investigations such as that in Pascagoula, and one in New Jersey's Raritan Bay, the CDC firmly defined the threat of polluted shellfish.

Perhaps the most novel CDC hepatitis detective work centered in West Branch, Michigan, a 2,000-soul hamlet where in 1968 close to sixty cases of infectious hepatitis surfaced during May. EIS officer Dr. Stephen C. Schoenbaum arrived from Atlanta to detect the source. Interviews with patients established several common eating places, particularly a bakery. With an associate from the EIS, Dr. E. Eugene Page, Jr., Schoenbaum spent a night observing the hired hands at the bakery. One of the employees had recovered from hepatitis earlier in the spring, but the two physicians were stumped when they saw that while there was literally hands-on work with the raw ingredients, the bread and pastry went into ovens at temperatures sufficient to destroy any hepatitis organisms. About ready to quit and look for new leads, Schoenbaum and Page watched at 3:30 a.m. as the one baker who had been sick removed the baked goods and began to apply glazes. To the epidemiologists' amazement and edification, he smeared the frostings on with his bare hands, without regard for sanitation. The mystery was instantly solved, the source of hepatitis identified.

Hepatitis is both pervasive and persistent. There are perhaps 200,000 Type B carriers in the U.S. alone—and 200 million worldwide. There are 80,000 to 100,000 cases of Type B in the U.S. annually. In fact, hepatitis is so widespread and is so threatening that there is a CDC unit in Phoenix exclusively devoted to research and control of this disease. It was natural for Verna Barefoot to expect to receive a high amount of expertise from the CDC.

When the EIS's Carl Armstrong arrived in New Bern from Virginia, he immediately visited the Craven County Hospital to examine and talk to the patients. "By the time I arrived, the local doctors knew that all four cases had been using drugs, injecting themselves. We needed to find the common links between them to locate the source of the disease. I managed to talk for a few minutes with Keller. He knew one of the other guys in the hospital but not the remaining two. Keller had used cocaine, he told me, three times, and he said the last use came when he was with a friend on May 15. He swore he took nothing intravenous since then. One problem with tracking hepatitis B is that it can have a long incubation period; it can be anywhere from five weeks to five months. So obviously it was difficult to pinpoint when Keller became infected. He was too sick to say much more." And indeed, Keller died within a few hours of speaking with Armstrong.

The medical reports on the remaining cases were not optimistic. "Ordinarily in hepatitis, there's pain from a swelling of the liver and you can feel it below the rib cage," explains Armstrong. "But in these cases the damage was incredible; it wasn't just a piece of the liver that was injured. The livers were just annihilated." And within a week, two more persons were dead and additional cases with the same lethal fulminant hepatitis were admitted to the hospital.

The hunt for the flash point of the infections required the two CDC investigators to operate with great sensitivity. To most people in New Bern, illegal drugs were associated with big cities like New York, Miami, and Chicago, and not with their small, bucolic city surrounded by farmland. "The local authorities were reluctant to accept that there was a drug problem," says Don Francis. "At the same time the pressure upon us was incredible. The newspapers, TV, and radio were after us every day and there was no way to hide. There was only one motel; they knew where to find us.

"We needed a lot of information about illegal activities. But also the local law-enforcement officials wanted to know if there had been foul play; if people had been killed either deliberately or accidentally by giving them bad drugs. The problem was to get information from the patients and other people who knew about the use of drugs without violating confidences or losing anyone's trust because they thought we would get them in trouble with the police."

Relationships among the interested parties often were strained. Craven County Sheriff Pete Bland said one day that his office was "following any leads they get," and that any information would be "kept confidential." He added, "We are working hand-in-glove with the health department. If this turns from a medical case into a criminal one, we are prepared for an investigation."

The public health authorities realized immediately that the sheriff's remarks could jeopardize their efforts to find people exposed to hepatitis. Dr. Verna Barefoot responded to Bland's statements, remarking that "hand-in-glove" meant only that the law-enforcement officials were not hampering the efforts of the CDC investigators. "If he [Bland] meant that we are collaborating with them, this has not been done. All our interviews are considered confidential."

The CDC investigators followed the same course. Says Francis, "Our tack was to stay away from the police, to leave the questioning about drug contacts to the local health people. We were able to advise the police that we didn't think anyone had intentionally poisoned drug users."

Meanwhile Craven County was in a near panic as the available information appeared in the press. "People aren't doing drugs right now because they're scared to death of it," said one person familiar with the New Bern drug scene. Those who had used drugs risked discovery of their abuse of narcotics by rushing to the hospital for examination. A woman who had recently snorted coke that seemed "good" nevertheless went for tests because of fear and broke down and cried when she showed signs (subsequently insignificant) of early stages of hepatitis. Another user said after a medical examination: "I did coke in the Bridgeton area and they [doctors] said, 'You know what's going on, don't you?' And I said I didn't want to catch hep and die."

The public health authorities mounted an intensive surveillance to find any more cases of hepatitis. Almost 300 people had had contact with the total of nine people now hospitalized. Fifty-four individuals admitted to using intravenous drugs, indicating that the drug problem in the New Bern area was not radically different from that observed in places more readily associated with narcotics.

There was friction between the press and segments of the community. Bobbie Golec was "not too thrilled" with newspaper reports, particularly those from out of the community, feeling that they sensationalized the material. The local *New Bern Sun Journal* carried an editorial noting that Craven County Hospital authorities had passed out false information about the gravity of the problem and then refused to provide the names of the sick. The *Sun Journal* noted how vital it was for the identities of the victims to be made public in order that any acquaintance could come forward, be tested, and protected against infection.

Verna Barefoot arranged for the health department offices to see people evenings and weekends in order to accommodate the large number of people who subsequently admitted to either knowing the patients, using drugs, or feeling ill from hepatitis-type symptoms.

The crucial point for the CDC team (and for the police) was the source of the drugs. The total of nine cases that entered the hospitals within a period of three weeks was composed of two entirely separate groups—one from New Bern, and the other from the community across the river, Bridgeton, where Keller had lived. Some members were from blue-collar backgrounds; others had come from families in the professions. Both groups patronized local night spots, but not the same ones. None of the nine appeared to be addicted; drug use was confined to weekends for "recreation."

Enterprising reporters from the *Sun Journal* were able to find local drug users and get them to talk freely. One woman offered a critique on the quality of narcotics being sold. "The coke offered me was nasty, trashy-looking." She told of house parties that went on at a trailer, the home of three young men who were involved in the drug traffic.

A man who claimed to have been a cocaine user for many years explained his taste test for the right stuff. "I put a bit on my tongue and it makes my tongue numb, if it's good stuff." He went on to report that recently "a fellow tried to sell me some. I tasted it and all it did was make my mouth bitter. I asked him what the hell was he trying to pass on me. Then

I washed my mouth out." The experienced users all described the local vendors as prone to cutting their products with a variety of substances.

"We began looking at all chemicals that can damage the liver, but there are so many, that might be involved, not just hard drugs," says Armstrong. "Based on the first four interviews it was looking for a needle in a haystack. We checked out where patients worked to see if anything in their occupations might have done the damage but found nothing." The investigators even considered the possibility of some potent wild mushrooms or a variety of herbal tea, but neither of these was consumed by the victims.

The outbreak in Craven County struck young adults; the two men with responsibility for finding the causes were not that much removed in age from the people they had come to help. Carl Armstrong, unlike some other EIS recruits, went straight from his undergraduate work at Kenyon in Ohio to medical school at Case Western Reserve in Cleveland. After an internship at Tufts New England Medical Center and a stint on the staff of the Brockton, Massachusetts, Hospital emergency room, Armstrong signed on with the CDC. "I'd always been fascinated with communicable diseases," says he, "but at the beginning of my career in medicine I was involved in a wide variety of medical problems. Then I read some articles by Berton Roueché [the *New Yorker* magazine writer on medical detection]. That pointed me toward the CDC."

As a young physician working in an emergency ward in a blue-collar town, Armstrong had been well aware of the violent acts of humanity. He saw his share of gunshot wounds, stabbings, and drug overdoses. Still, he confesses, "The New Bern experience was a real eye-opener. They weren't addicts but lads who held good jobs. They had no needle tracks on their arms. The community was shocked, but the use of drugs was widespread."

Don Francis undoubtedly had more of a sense of the ambience in the subterranean drug scene of Craven County. He had done his undergraduate work at the University of California at Berkeley just as the so-called counterculture blossomed there. After medical school at Northwestern, he interned at the Los Angeles County Medical Center of the University of Southern California. As an intern he confronted the military draft. "I had been active in the antiwar movement," remembers Francis, "and everybody was aware I was up to my ears in politics. I had declared myself a conscientious objector, but the way things worked the draft board would not accept an application as a CO until you were called. And once you were classified 1-A, if you went to Canada you were facing criminal charges. I had made up my mind to go over the border, and I asked Paul Wehrle, who was the chief physician in the pediatric section of the medical center, for some advice on practicing pediatrics in Canada. He asked me why I wanted to know, and when I told him, Wehrle, who'd been an EIS officer in the first class of 1951, told me about the CDC." Thus, the Vietnam War guided another permanent asset to the CDC.

After his tour in the EIS (he was part of the same class as David Fraser), Francis worked as a member of the World Health Organization teams on efforts to stamp out smallpox in the Sudan, Yugoslavia, India, and Bangladesh, before assignment to the Phoenix hepatitis center.

The screening of blood from the contacts turned up twenty-five individuals with some marker of a hepatitis B infection. For most of them it only meant that they had the disease, but one, a 25-year-old, Howard Yancy (pseudonym), not only carried Type B in his blood but also was the brother of Sally Yancy (pseudonym), a young woman fighting for her life in Craven County Hospital.

Carl Armstrong actually had questioned Sally Yancy. "She denied ever using any intravenous drugs," says Armstrong. "I talked to her several times and she stuck to that story, and then she deteriorated, went into a coma. Her friends and her brother came and told the health department, 'Look, she didn't tell the truth. She did use drugs.'"

Sally and Howard Yancy had a sister; she too tested out as positive for having had a hepatitis infection, although in her case she was not a carrier. The pieces began to fall into place. Howard Yancy was apparently the one person who moved between the two distinct social groups that had developed the disease. "When you're watching your sister die," remarks Carl Armstrong, "you don't hold back information." Yancy was what might be described as an intermediate-level drug supplier. Not a dealer himself, it was through him and at his living quarters that the young people of Craven County obtained drugs and shot up.

Howard Yancy admitted not only to playing the role of a middleman in local drug use but also to sharing needles with visitors to his home. "A lot of these youngsters," observes Armstrong, "were afraid to take any drug apparatus home with them, so they used it at his place." Their fear of parental outrage and discovery led them into jeopardy.

The establishment of Yancy as the link to the victims explained only part of the mystery. Still in question was why the disease had been so lethal. Discarded almost immediately were the candidates such as wild mushrooms or herbal teas that might somehow have stimulated the infection to greater virulence. The obvious conclusion was that drugs in combination with hepatitis were what had triggered the fulminant character of the disease. "Through a local public health service officer," says Francis, "we arranged to buy some cocaine. The deal was done at gunpoint—I was glad that I did not have to participate—and for $85 we bought one gram. Lab analysis showed that it was $85 worth of No-Doz and lidocaine. The lidocaine when put on the tongue gives it a tingle the way cocaine is supposed to do. You can get these drugs easily. No-Doz is just some caffeine available in any pharmacy. They all told us they were using cocaine; but if our sample was any evidence they were getting caffeine and lidocaine, stuff you can buy in any pharmacy. The problem, of course, in testing any illegal substance is you never can tell the quality of one batch from the next. Furthermore, the people who use it don't know what they're getting either." The investigators also scored a capsule of RJ-8, allegedly an amphetamine. Lab inspection proved it was only caffeine and a "Black Beauty"; another pill labeled an upper was just more caffeine.

There is no evidence in the literature that cocaine does turn an ordinary hepatitis infection into a more ferocious sickness. However, those who were sick, including cases able to talk before they died, professed to taking another drug along with their "cocaine." This was a substance called MDA or methylene dioxyamphetamine. It is a poor man's upper, a cheap version of speed, manufactured locally. All seven of the ful-

minant cases hospitalized claimed to have injected MDA
along with the cocaine. (Two other hospitalized individuals
with a hepatitis B infection were classified as nonfulminant.)

The investigators obtained samples of the MDA available
in New Bern. A light, brownish powder, when used intra-
venously, it supposedly brought on a warm euphoria without
hallucinations. The experiences of users, however, varied
widely, most likely because quality control was not the rule
for MDA production any more than for the local cocaine.
Drug dealers confessed to cutting MDA with sugar and a
hot-chocolate mix. On the other hand, the investigators were
able to buy four different samples of what was labeled MDA
and analysis showed it to be what was advertised.

The hullabaloo over the epidemic and the various investigations coincided with the end of the New Bern epidemic. The
publicity undoubtedly scared some individuals away from
narcotics abuse; those who continued more than likely became
far more careful once they learned how deadly contaminated
needles could be.

Don Francis pursued the question of why the disease had
been the fulminating kind in laboratory experiments. MDA
had previously been shown to affect the central nervous system of mice and humans but not the liver. "We gave two
chimps the New Bern strain of Type B and injected them with
large amounts of the MDA. One animal died the next day,
but not of fulminant hepatitis. The other chimp ran the normal course of hepatitis B. We did other experiments with
MDA and hepatitis and could not find any relationship. Of
course, one problem remains: Whether the substance we got
was the same that the victims received.

"There was a second theory—that some new, more virulent
superstrain of hepatitis B was present at New Bern. Again
we infected some chimps with the sera from New Bern and
the chimps got mildly sick, nothing like what had happened to
the people in North Carolina. That seems to rule out any
superstrain.

"We're still struggling with a third possibility. The sister
who survived [Alice Yancy] had Non-A, Non-B, and her
boyfriend had Type B. Possibly the victims developed both
B and Non-A, Non-B simultaneously. We're seeing something like this in an outbreak in Venezuela among a group

of Indians. There's an additional ingredient, something we call the Delta factor, that seems to have been seen occasionally before in the Amazon River Basin in the middle 1960s."

Ordinarily outsiders, particularly those from the federal government, do not find favor in small communities such as New Bern. But recalling those days, Verna Barefoot says, "I was impressed by the swiftness of the CDC's response and the dedication with which they worked with families. They were remarkably sensitive to the feelings of people."

With the end of his EIS tour, Armstrong stayed on in Virginia, taking a fellowship in infectious diseases at the Medical College of Virginia Hospitals.

Francis continued to supervise research that might unravel the tangle of the Craven County epidemic, although it is unlikely that research directly connected with that affair will lead to a definitive finding. Instead, Francis believes, the Venezuelan outbreak and the mysterious Delta factor may provide the vital clues. "Working with the EIS was fun; it's really only because of the absence of an EIS officer at the time of the North Carolina epidemic that I got to go out into the field. I miss that kind of work but I recognize that I'm at a level where you can't just go off."

Craven County, meanwhile, has seen no new outbreak of fulminant hepatitis; presumably substance abusers continue in their old ways, although perhaps with more sophistication about hypodermic needles, like the doctor discovered by Bruce Dull in New Jersey.

8

A Winter's Tale of a Summer Disease

THE SICKNESS begins a few hours after a meal with a growing feeling of malaise. Then come the increasingly painful sharp pains in the stomach—cramps. A spate of diarrhea follows, but the conditions may not be relieved. There is an incessant queasiness, a nausea that makes even the thought of food repellent, and frequently one says, "It must have been something I ate."

The gut-wrenching agony that follows a meal is not the result of poisonous food but rather of a devilish kind of bacteria known as salmonella that has found its way into food or drink and then multiplied at astronomical rates in the intestinal tract. Salmonella poisoning is the unwanted guest at a church supper, the unexpected hangover from a picnic, and the nightmare of all food processors and restaurateurs. Most commonly, a salmonella attack fells dozens of people who have attended the same function, dined in the same restaurant, or bought from the same vendor.

Salmonella draws its name from its Americn discoverer, veterinarian Daniel Salmon. The label covers 1,800 different strains of bacteria with similar characteristics. (In addition, there are a number of other bacteria species such as gardia and shigella that may raise havoc in the stomach.) Salmonella's effects may range from nothing more than a vague gastrointestinal upset all the way to a life-threatening depletion of bodily fluids. (Included in the 1,800 varieties of salmonella is typhoid fever.) Some types are pathogenic for both animals and humans; others threaten only mankind, which means that a raiser of livestock may be unaware that the animals he markets could be diseased. Salmonellas are identified by name based upon the place where the particular kind was first isolated—*Salmonella cubana, Salmonella newport, Salmonella newbrunswick, Salmonella waycross* (Georgia).

Infection can come from contact with animals that harbor the bacteria, from fecal contamination of food or water, or from human carriers who have picked up the organisms on their hands and then handle food served to people. The CDC hears of perhaps fifty epidemic attacks annually (thousands of Americans are victims every year). In a memorable investigation of a salmonella epidemic that struck 1,600 people in the California city of Riverside, the CDC investigators discovered the bacteria lurking in a unit of the city's water-supply system. When that section was shut down, so was the epidemic, evoking the shade of John Snow more than a century after his triumph with the Broad Street pump.

Beginning in mid-December 1980 and persisting for a period of better than eight weeks, hospital authorities in Steubenville, Ohio, became aware of a sharp increase in the number of people presenting themselves at emergency rooms with severe stomach cramps, diarrhea, even blood in their stools. The most severely affected spent from three to five days in the hopsital before they recovered. Treatment consisted usually of intravenous feedings with a saline solution that contained dextrose to redress the drastic dehydration resulting from the severe diarrhea.

The public health authorities had little difficulty in identifying the culprit—*Salmonella muenchen* (for Munich)—but they were stumped when it came to locating the source of the bacteria. On January 28, 1982, the Ohio State Office of Epidemiology placed a call to the CDC in Atlanta. EIS officer Dr. David N. Taylor of the Enteric Disease Branch (headed by Paul Blake, who conducted the cholera investigations discussed in Chapter 3) and Dr. Roger A. Feldman, acting director of the Bacterial Disease Division, discussed the situation.

Subsequently, the CDC officials also chatted with the authorities in Weirton, West Virginia, which is just across the river from Steubenville, and learned that the acute-care hospital in that city had also witnessed a dramatic rise in the number of people being treated there for *Salmonella muenchen* infections.

On January 29, Taylor and Emmett V. Schmidt, then a Ph.D. in epidemiology on a two-month fellowship at the CDC, traveled to Steubenville. Taylor says, "While I was at Harvard Medical School and during my internship and residencies in Buffalo and at Johns Hopkins I became interested in tropical medicine. Then I went to the London School of Hygiene and Tropical Medicine for further study. While I was a research fellow in Panama I met Rob Ryder, who'd been in the EIS, and he talked up that program as a way to really understand epidemiology."

Emmett Schmidt's route to Steubenville was somewhat different. "As an undergraduate at Harvard I planned to go into pure research," says the ebullient Schmidt. "I was interested in physiology but the more I thought about it the more I realized that studying what happens to a human being on a treadmill is not a good way to survive in this world. So I decided to see if I could combine medicine and research, taking care of patients as well as doing scientific investigations."

To combine his interests, Schmidt first secured his Ph.D. in epidemiology and then pursued an M.D. degree. As a medical student he leaped at an opportunity for the two-month tour with the EIS. "I am a great fan of Berton Roueché [the author of innumerable pieces on epidemiology for the *New Yorker* magazine] and I suppose subliminally that turned me on to the work of the CDC."

Before he was dispatched to Ohio, Schmidt worked on the problem of necrotizing enterocolitis (a breakdown of intestinal tissue) among newborn babies. "It was something that had not been seen before medicine was able to help premature infants survive," remarks Schmidt, "and the infection was confined to nurseries." However, Schmidt spent most of his career at the CDC in Steubenville.

When the pair of CDC investigators arrived in Steubenville, they conferred with the state and local health authorities. But the officials could add nothing more than the latest statistics. Taylor and Schmidt next sought out some of the victims who continued to show up at hospital emergency rooms in Steubenville and across the river.

"Usually, in a salmonella outbreak," explains Taylor, "everyone gets sick at the same time—they've all been to the same church supper and eaten the same contaminated potato salad. If you were to plot the epidemic on a graph it would consist of a curve that is flat at the start, peaks in the middle, and then becomes flat again. But that wasn't the way the epidemic was in Steubenville. Instead of a peak pinpointing one meal or a single day, the epidemic was erratic. Cases continued to crop up, day after day. You couldn't tie the epidemic to any single event."

The investigators considered the possibility that it was another Riverside. They plotted the cases on a map. That eliminated the water supply as a suspect. "The cases were in different townships with different water sources," says Taylor.

"Because it was that time of the year," says Taylor, "we started to wonder about holiday food. From talking to the patients and the local authorities we knew there were no common links among the victims; they didn't all use the same parmesan cheese at Joe's Pizza Parlor. In fact, they weren't from the same social groups; some of the victims were high school students, others steel-mill workers, and there were a lot of very young kids. But it was possible that some kind of traditional holiday food was consumed by all of them. One good candidate was chocolate; it's been frequently associated with salmonella outbreaks and it's a common holiday food. But we couldn't find any indications of the bacteria in chocolate sold in stories or supermarkets." Following the holiday-treat line of reasoning, Taylor and Schmidt also checked into cheeses, dressings, spices, and even fruitcakes. None of these items could be connected to the illness.

The epidemiologists then focused upon another specific food, ham. "The ethnic background in Steubenville," explains Taylor, "was such that instead of turkey, many people ate ham for the holidays. We canvassed the stores, testing what they sold, trying to find any supplier or food handler who might himself have been sick and then transmitted the bacteria to the meat which was distributed through the area." Again, the investigators came to a dead end. They could not tie either fresh meats or processed tins of ham to the epidemic. "Many people had eaten ham," says Taylor, "but it either wasn't purchased in the same store or else it was a different brand."

"I was really sold on the holiday-foods notion," says Schmidt. "The idea of ham for the holidays was strange to me, but that gave the possibility even more credence." Schmidt was aware that *Salmonella st. paul* had infected precooked roast beef and ham from a Philadelphia food processor. *Salmonella chester* and *Salmonella tennessee* were discovered in patients who dined on rare roast beef supplied by an Albany, New York, vendor. These outbreaks occurred in the late '70s. Nevertheless the meat suspect was exonerated. The CDC agents next considered the high proportion of young children who had become ill and scrutinized baby foods. They found no evidence of contaminated baby food.

"We kept going back to a couple of things," recalls Taylor. "The first was that such a high percentage of the patients were either young adults, 20 to 29, or else kids under four. But we couldn't find a common denominator for even the same age groups. A lot of them knew each other from high school but they did not hang out together. The children were not from a single day-care center or area where they played together.

"The other thing was the way the cases kept occurring. Even while we were in Steubenville, they trickled into the hospital." Adding to the mystery, epidemics of *Salmonella muenchen* are more commonly seen during the summer than winter. The particular bacterial strain grows better at higher temperatures.

"Toward the end of our first week, we were fairly well convinced that we hadn't missed anything in the way of stores, restaurants, or food," says Taylor, "but we continued to check out places. One day, Emmett and I were with a sanitation officer looking at the ham in a supermarket when we noticed a young woman. She appeared distraught, her eye makeup was running; she was either drunk or strung out on pills. The sanitarian remarked to us that drugs were being recognized as an important problem in the area. There was a lot of unemployment; Steubenville and the surrounding communities like Weirton were extremely depressed economically and emotionally, favorable conditions for drug use. It was also another good reason to stop thinking about restaurants; the local people couldn't afford to eat out that much."

The possibilities that salmonella might be connected with drug use was not farfetched. Taylor knew of a report on some capsules which bore a dye designed to trace the workings of the digestive system. Somehow they became contaminated with *Salmonella cubana* organisms, resulting in an epidemic among those who received the pills.

The investigators went back to the people who had been victims of the epidemic. "None of them would admit to using hard drugs," says Taylor. "It's a very conservative place; a high school student who admitted to smoking pot would be expelled. It was only from a high school counselor that we could learn a bit about the extent of drug use. No one admitted using anything. After all, not only was this a pretty conservative area, but also we were federal agents, of a sort, asking about drugs."

The possibility that the infection might have a tie-in with the use of illegal drugs was already stirring in the back of Schmidt's mind when he was offered a lead from an unexpected source, his wife, Deborah. She was living in North Carolina while he was engaged in the Steubenville investigation, and she was rather anxious for her husband to complete his work and return. During a telephone call to his wife, Schmidt described the lack of progress in the investigation and the odd features of the infection, including the strange concentration of the population at risk. Deborah Schmidt, who had been turned on to Berton Roueché by her husband, and who was reading the writer's *Eleven Blue Men*, suggested one common substance among people that age, marijuana.

Even as Taylor and Schmidt speculated on the possibility that drugs might be involved, they came across a phenomenon that piqued their curiosity. Betty Sanderson (pseudonym) was a young woman whose child had suffered a severe *Salmonella muenchen* attack. The youngster had recovered after treatment. As a matter of routine, however, the members of the family were tested for salmonella organisms in their systems. Although Mrs. Sanderson had not been sick, she tested positive for having the bacteria in her body. She continued to show signs of it for a number of weeks. (Not everybody infected with salmonella becomes violently ill; some people suffer only a mild stomach upset, and others may not have any discomfort.) What was peculiar in this instance was that Betty Sanderson had abruptly stopped passing salmonella in her stool.

"We questioned her," says Schmidt, "and asked her what had happened that was different. She informed us that she had become pregnant." That was of interest to the Sandersons, but the condition does not confer immunity to salmonella.

"We asked her if she was eating differently, doing anything different," says Taylor, "and after some questioning she admitted that because she was pregnant she had stopped smoking marijuana."

Her information sent the investigators after the households where the disease had been diagnosed. Five people between the ages of 10 and 39 finally admitted to use of marijuana, while another seven people admitted to "close contact"— that is, being in a room with others who had been smoking pot.

From three households where *Salmonella muenchen* had appeared, the CDC investigators obtained samples of marijuana. Every one of these contained the bacteria responsible for the epidemic. Significantly, the pot had been purchased at different times and the dealers were not the same individuals. Obviously a shipment of marijuana to the Steubenville area was contaminated.

"Salmonella via pot had never been found before," says Taylor (although one historic investigation by the CDC discovered that the dizziness, muscular weakness, vomiting, and blurred vision of nine people at a Colorado office party came from marijuana in a cake). "The samples we tested in Steubenville not only were positive for salmonella," says Taylor, "but the contamination also was very heavy."

Unlike Don Francis and the others seeking clues to hepatitis in New Bern (see Chapter 7), Taylor and company did not have to buy drugs on the street. "While they may have been nervous about admitting to drug use to federal agents such as ourselves," says Taylor, "the people had suffered enough from the illness to want the matter cleared up. We were also very careful to ensure that the names of people we talked to never were disclosed to the local police."

Still, it was an unusual situation. "If it had been a contaminated ham or some other food," remarks Taylor, "we would call the FDA and say, 'Please recall this product.' With pot you obviously cannot do that. We did go public with our findings, and we interviewed everyone who had been found to harbor salmonella and explained the situation. We convinced them that we weren't going to prosecute anyone. Half of the people who were sick were kids. You certainly weren't going to prosecute them. Furthermore, many of the cases were people who said they were around someone smoking marijuana, and that's not illegal. Unfortunately, you can become infected from a person who is smoking contaminated pot; he or she is, in effect, a carrier."

There was no pressure for action by local authorities. "When we informed the city health commissioner that the source of the epidemic was contaminated marijuana, he fell off his chair. He couldn't believe it," says Taylor.

Taylor and Schmidt had put together a highly plausible source for the outbreak in Steubenville, but, points out Taylor, "The CDC has sometimes been criticized for using the results of an investigation as proof of a hypothesis which itself is created by the facts of that investigation. Ideally you need an entirely separate epidemic to prove your point."

As a matter of fact, at the very same time that Taylor and Schmidt were hunting down the cause in Steubenville, twenty-seven cases of *Salmonella muenchen* had been isolated in the Michigan towns of Lansing and Owosso. With the data from Ohio in hand, David Taylor trekked to Michigan (Schmidt's term with the CDC had expired). "They were also blue-collar people, the same age roughly as in Ohio, but they were not as conservative. Actually they were quite forthcoming. We had no difficulty in finding out about the use of marijuana. And when we tested the samples we again isolated *Salmonella muenchen*."

In an official EIS report and subsequently in a paper in the *New England Medical Journal*, Taylor and Schmidt traced the epidemiological pathways for a marijuana-based epidemic of salmonella. They reported that the Drug Enforcement Agency (DEA) estimates about 93 percent of the marijuana consumed in the United States is imported from Colombia and Jamaica. U.S. crops are usually sold and used in the state where grown. Marijuana which is shipped into the United States is stored in the country of origin at room temperature in a dry atmosphere. Contamination of the product with salmonella may occur because the producers use animal feces for fertilization, because of inadvertent introduction of bacteria during drying and storage, or simply through the direct adulteration of the pot with dried animal manure in order to increase the weight of the marijuana.

When stored at room temperature, salmonella remain viable but do not multiply. However, rolling a cigarette with the contaminated pot may easly transfer bacteria to a person's fingers, providing a way for the salmonella to find its way directly into the individual's mouth or onto the food he or she handles. Of course, once the cigarette is placed in the mouth, the organisms are in a position to invade the intestinal tract, where their numbers multiply rapidly. Conceivably, salmonella may even be inhaled into the lungs by a person smoking contaminated pot, but Taylor and Schmidt detected no evidence of this happening.

Heavy users of marijuana have reduced stomach acidity. Indeed, experiments have shown them more vulnerable to cholera for that reason. Conceivably the use of the drug in Steubenville may have cut stomach acidity enough to enhance the ability of the salmonella to survive. Regular tobacco cigarettes do not inhibit the manufacture of stomach acid.

The marijuana findings explained the concentration of sickness among young adults, but what about the excessive number of cases among very young children? They do not use the drug. However, their parents and their elder siblings who fed them passed salmonella via their fingers that had been contaminated from the pot. Salmonella infections of young children frequently are quite severe, and also, in the eyes of parents, more threatening. As a consequence, youngsters are more likely to be brought for medical treatment after an attack than adults or even older children. Based on this experience. Taylor suggests that investigators of salmonella-type epidemics among kids might be well advised to look into the habits of their parents or siblings for an explanation of an outbreak that on the surface seems limited to young children.

To confirm the discoveries of Taylor and Schmidt further, investigations into salmonella epidemics in Georgia and Alabama revealed the same pattern of pot use among the victims and their kin.

Emmett Schmidt completed medical school—"the best part of it was the two months with the CDC." He accepted a pediatrics residency at the Boston Children's Hospital. "There's still a chance I'll go into some kind of epidemiology," muses Schmidt. "My career is still evolving."

David Taylor held a brief reunion with the Schmidts in Boston in the spring of 1982 after he was sent there to look into another epidemic of gastrointestinal disease. "Deborah Schmidt had an idea about this case too," says Taylor. "She suggested that it might be the Easter flowers that had become contaminated. However, we couldn't find any proof of that."

Taylor's term at the CDC ended in 1982. At the time he said, "I tried to find a job where I could still do investigative epidemiology." He succeeded, becoming one of the rare EIS alumni who not only managed to continue his role as a disease detective, but also moved in an opposite path to that of many EIS officers. Taylor went into the U.S. Army, to serve with a unit in Bangkok, checking into diseases that might threaten American military units.

The investigations of both the hepatitis outbreak in New Bern and the epidemic in Steubenville point up several more critical aspects to the traffic in illegal substances. Because illegal drugs are of necessity processed without controls that prevent adulteration or contamination, the potential consequences from drug use go far beyond those inherent in abuse of the substances. And because sale of dope is against the law the work of investigators into epidemics can be substantially more difficult.

CHAPTER
9

The Curse of the Swineherd

EARLY IN JUNE 1971, Harold and Martha Wilson (pseudonym), along with their four children, Arthur, 18, Donald, 14, Mary, 13, and John, 9, left their home in central Oregon bent on an ambitious three-month exploration of the United States. Packed into a camper, they headed east, spending their nights sleeping under the star-filled skies that roof the national parks, cooling themselves by day with swims in the lakes that dotted the route and driving several hundred miles a day during the sun-lit hours.

By June 13 they were in Renville, Minnesota, 100 miles east of Minneapolis, for what was to be a highlight of the trek, a gathering of the family clan. The reunion marked the high school graduation of the eldest son of Jason and Sarah Cox; Sarah was Martha Wilson's sister. Kin from around the country had traveled to the Renville pig farm. Altogether the congregation brought together nine families—grandparents, mothers, fathers, aunts, uncles, nieces, nephews, cousins, and assorted in-laws—totaling forty-one people.

Several families contributed to a buffet feast of cold baked ham, turkey, Jell-O, tossed green salad, and an abundance of cookies and candies. The celebrants slaked their thirst with hot coffee and Kool-Aid, mixing the powdered drink with the clear, cold water of the Cox well. It was a glorious occasion, the adults sitting and reminiscing while the youngsters darted about the farm past chicken runs and pigpens to churn around a muddy, meandering track aboard go-carts. In between rides and games, the muddy-handed kids constantly returned to the tables for food and drink.

When the partying was over, the Wilsons took to the road

again, pausing for nights in campgrounds and sampling the waters along their route. It was in Rhode Island, nearly three weeks after they left Oregon, that the idyl turned into a nightmare. The first victim was 14-year-old Donald. He complained of sore muscles and a headache and seemed unable to keep food down. Initially, Donald's parents figured their son had picked up a touch of flu and thought they could ride out his discomfort with over-the-counter medicines. But in quick succession, Arthur and then his brother John and finally even sister Mary developed similar symptoms. At this point, the Wilsons decided to bring their brood to the attention of a physician. Of the four children, Donald was in the worst condition. He was feverish, his joints and muscles pained him, and his continued vomiting had dehydrated him. Taking no chances, the doctor arranged for all four children to be hospitalized while an attempt was made to ascertain the nature of their illness.

The staff at the hospital tapped fluid from the spinal columns of the Wilson kids and subjected blood and urine specimens to microscopic study. The preliminary diagnosis for Donald and his siblings was aseptic meningitis, an inflammation of the membranes in the central nervous system but without the presence of any gross signs of a bacterial infection such as pus. As the most severely affected, Donald received an antibiotic; the others were kept in bed and their conditions were monitored. Almost as suddenly as the mysterious disease had struck it disappeared. The children all recovered in a few days and were discharged from the hospital.

In the laboratory, the technicians observed a highly unusual organism in the specimens taken from the Wilson kids. It was a leptospire, a kind of spirochete—a spiral-shaped bacterium—known as *Leptospirosa autumnalis*. Leptospirosis is a zoonosis, a disease transmittable to humans from animals, a characteristic that caused the malady to be labeled "swineherd's disease" at one point in history. In its most serious human manifestation, as Weil's disease, it can devastate the central nervous system, and although the outbreaks are quite rare and sometimes asymptomatic, leptospirosis can be responsible for meningitis, hepatitis, and nephritis (kidney disorder).

Because the ailment is so rarely seen, the authorities in Rhode Island were quite concerned about how the Wilson children had contracted the disease. However, upon the recovery of the children, the family piled back into their camper and reembarked upon their journey, leaving the mystery behind them, temporarily.

In October of that same year the Wilsons, back in Oregon, received a telephone call from the EIS officer assigned to the state health department. He happened to be Dr. Donald Francis, the same individual who subsequently became an expert in hepatitis and headed the investigation into the occurrence of the disease in New Bern, North Carolina (Chapter 7).

"We were notified by the authorities in Rhode Island," remembered Francis several years later. "The people in New England had been quite perplexed by the experiences of the Wilsons and they thought it prudent that someone pursue the matter in an effort to find out how the children caught the disease. After I called the family, I arranged to drive down to see them.

"The more I talked to them, the more discouraged I became. From the time they started their trip until the kids became sick they had stopped off in so many different places, swum in so many different bodies of water, that it would be a monumental job to find out where they became infected. There was no guarantee that the organisms were even still at the site."

The net result of the interview after several hours was largely frustration for Francis. "I was literally putting on my jacket, taking it from the back of the chair as I was about to leave, when I asked them if they had had any problems with mosquitoes. Bites from mosquitoes, particularly if the person scratches them enough, provide an easy entry for leptospires. The answer was yes, that they had indeed been plagued by mosquitoes at the campgrounds and the kids in particular had been bitten heavily. Then I asked another question, even though I was still preparing to leave. I wanted to know if they had come in contact with any substantial amounts of mud during their travels. Animal dropping and urine often leave leptospires in mud, and if a person gets the mud on his body that can be a means of infection. Oh yes, they all remembered. It had rained considerably just before the big reunion in Renville, Minnesota. They all had managed to get mud on their bodies as a result."

Francis now put down his jacket to ask the critical question. "Do you know if anyone else who was at that family get-together was sick?" The answer was again affirmative. The Wilsons had heard from their relatives that a number of people had been sick shortly afterward, but everyone assumed that there was some kind of flu going around, and no one in Minnesota was so sick that hospitalization was required.

Francis decided that the only way to confirm his suspicion that a leptospirosis epidemic had occurred at Renville would be through testing of everyone who attended the party. He received permission from his superiors to fly to the Midwest and visit the Cox farm at Renville.

"I learned that eleven more people had become sick after the party, making a total of fifteen out of the forty-one who attended. The disease had showed up anywhere from sixteen to twenty-six days following the reunion. That was within the known incubation period of leptospirosis. In addition to these individuals, most of whom had significant levels of antibodies for leptospirosis, three more people who did not exhibit any symptoms of illness, nevertheless, when tested, showed elevated antibody activity. Actually, those who had been sick but did not have any antibody reaction had been treated with penicillin, which is known to inhibit any serological conversion in leptospirosis cases."

Francis pored over his known facts, looking for clues that would pinpoint the route taken by the infection. It was obvious that the disease was much more prevalent among children, with an attack rate of 67 percent in those under 15. More boys than girls had come down sick. On the surface it seemed as if all the children enjoyed the same opportunity for having mud with leptospires splashed upon them. But talking to the Cox family and recalling his discussions with the Wilsons, Francis zeroed in on the one activity that appeared to be a major factor, the rides on the go-carts.

The vehicles were fenderless, and the track laid out on the Cox farm wound through muddy paths past the barn and pigpen and disappeared into a portion of a nearby forest before bringing the riders back to the farm property.

"The kids were the ones who did most of the riding, particularly the boys," says Francis. "Furthermore, most of the children had cuts, bruises, abrasions, or mosquito bites—breaks in the skin." With the carts throwing up plenty of mud on the exposed parts of the body the youngsters were naturally quite open to infection. As if that were not enough, many of the children did not bother to clean off their muddy hands and fingers when they returned to the tables for their periodic raids upon the cookies and candies. Only one child who had been sick did not remember being liberally doused with mud.

Francis wondered why Donald Wilson, the 14-year-old, had been so severely infected. He questioned the child more and learned that on his ride mud had gotten into his eyes and onto his lips, and he also had a great many scratches on his mud-spattered arms, all of which probably led to his more extreme case. The EIS officer also was curious about the experience of the only adult woman who had come down with the disease. She had not ridden a go-cart. "However," says Francis, "she told me that after the family left the Cox farm, she had washed the mud from her son's body. She herself had a number of mosquito bites on her arms and hands and was vulnerable to the infection."

By the time Francis arrived in Renville, much of the livestock that had been on the farm back in June had been marketed. Only a number of brood sows remained. When tested they were negative for leptospires. It was possible that the animals that harbored the bacteria were among the pigs sold. In any event, the disease is not confined to domestic animals. Surveys by veterinarians in the Midwest have found infections in deer, and Francis noted that the track taken by the go-carts included a run along a muddy path through the forest where any number of fauna might have deposited a spoor packed with leptospires.

Even though the EIS officer detected a much higher attack rate for the disease among those who had come in close contact with the go-cart rides than among those who had not, one case seemed to confirm his thesis. A 16-year-old boy, a neighbor of the Coxes, had not attended the reunion. However, the evening after that event, he had visited the farm. "He was there only about ten minutes," says Francis, "but he spent most of that time scraping mud off a go-cart with a putty knife. He had open lesions on his hands from excoriated insect bites, and eight days later he became ill, showing the same symptoms as the others. When we tested his antibody reaction, it was positive."

Donald Francis's investigation into a leptospirosis epidemic reached a tidy conclusion, but diagnosis of the disease is difficult. "The symptoms are flu-like," says Francis, "and it could be easily overlooked in a human. Any number of people might be classified as a 'viral syndrome' or flu victims when in reality they've picked up leptospirosis."

Indeed, three years later, two workers at the Birmingham, Alabama, zoo developed serious respiratory infections. Physicians could not decide whether the animal attendants had meningitis, flu, or some other disease. Fearful of a possible epidemic that might strike the 400,000 zoo visitors to the zoo each year and the possible consequences for other employees, the state epidemiologists asked for CDC help. A two-man epidemiology team, veterinarians James G. Geistfeld and Daniel C. Anderson, investigated. Because they were familiar with zoonoses, the pair thought of leptospirosis. Their hunch proved true; a polar bear cub handled by the two sick men indeed had leptospirosis.

Just as Francis predicted, doctors, unfamiliar with the possibilities of a zoonosis, had missed the identity of the disease.

CHAPTER
10

Hemorrhagic Fevers

ON SEPTEMBER 23, 1976, Sister Marie Jean (pseudonym), awoke in the compound of the Roman Catholic mission at Yambuku, a small village set in the fetid Zairian rain forest. The Belgian nursing nun had been laboring long hours caring for people of the region afflicted with a mysterious malignant fever. On this particular morning, Sister Marie Jean felt hot herself and her head ached fiercely. She managed to walk the few steps to the 120-bed hospital which gave Yambuku a unique identity among the scattered settlements of the area.

The marauder of the Yambuku region resembled a familiar native threat, yellow fever. But the scourge ordinarily lacked the malevolence demonstrated by the current epidemic.

At the Yambuku hospital, alarmed by Marie Jean's sickness, her colleagues immediately bedded her down. Meanwhile, they continued the frantic struggle to cope with the fever that had already killed more than a hundred people. Local paramedical personnel continued to believe the problem was either typhoid or yellow fever.

Two days later, a pair of Zairian doctors flew into Yambuku from the capital city of Kinshasa for a firsthand view of the epidemic. Appalled by the savagery of the disease and the inability of the missionary hospital to control it, they quickly retreated to Kinshasa, taking with them the desperately ill Sister Marie Jean, another nursing nun, and a priest. The sick woman was placed in an isolated ward of Ngaliema Hospital, a small private institution.

By now Sister Marie Jean's temperature hovered steadily around 103° and her head pain was relentless. Unable to eat, she vomited frequently. Tiny spots dotted the inside of her mouth and her eyes. Aspirin brought no relief from the searing fever. Massive doses of antibiotics had no effect. Intravenous fluids and blood transfusions could not compensate for her ever-increasing dehydration. On the seventh day of her sickness, blood oozed from her gums. By the following morning she was bleeding from other orifices. Sister Marie Jean died only eight days after becoming ill.

Some 5,000 miles away, at the CDC in Atlanta, Dr. Karl Johnson, then chief of the Special Pathogens Branch, a man with almost twenty years of experience with the exotic diseases of the tropics, was engaged in routine lab work. He was totally unaware of the Zairian epidemic. "I received a telephone call from Hamburg," recalls the tall, earthy Johnson. "I didn't know the guy and why he came to me I'm not quite sure, except there was a mutual acquaintance, a virologist in Hamburg. Anyway, this fellow told me that he'd just been informed by a German roadbuilding crew in southern Sudan of an unidentified disease that was raging through the area around the town of Maridi. People were dying right and left. The hospital run by Caritas [a Catholic charity] there had closed. The staff either became sick and died or else left. None of the Europeans had caught it yet, but they were going to get the hell out of there as soon as possible. Everything was totally out of control.

"It was all news to us. When the doctor asked me what we were going to do about it I explained that there wasn't anything the CDC could do unless there was a request through the U.S. embassy or from the World Health Organization. I turned it around and asked him if he'd been in touch with WHO and what he was going to do about it."

The German physician answered that the health experts in his country had very little experience in this sort of thing. Johnson then alerted the international ears of the CDC to the epidemic. Confirmation of the outbreak filtered back from Khartoum and Juba, the principal cities of Sudan.

Johnson suspected the killer was a form of hemorrhagic virus. Confined largely to the tropical climes, these are the deadliest kinds of diseases known to modern medicine. The viruses destroy small blood vessels, causing internal bleeding, and, according to Johnson, "the person dies of irreversible shock." Only untreated rabies brings a higher fatality rate, and the viruses remain impervious to antibiotics. The information was sketchy, but one listening post also picked up word of the sinister events in Zaire.

Karl Johnson's acquaintance with the hemorrhagic viruses was more than the cool detachment of a curious scientist. He originally pursued medicine from a somewhat unusual ideological angle. "I was studying botany as an undergraduate at Oberlin during the Korean War. Then when MacArthur decided to take it to North Korea and the Chinese entered, we had a lot of bull sessions. I felt guilty as friends on campus were drafted. It looked like the war would last for twenty years and it didn't have much room for botanists. I decided to get in on the war by becoming a doctor."

By the time he completed medical school, peace reigned and Johnson had discovered microbiology. No longer motivated by the need to get in on the war, he fulfilled his military obligation through the National Institutes of Health. "There was an opening for field service in Panama," says Johnson. "Nobody else wanted to go, but I thought I'd see a bit of the world. My two-year term in Panama turned into thirteen fascinating years."

During this period Johnson had his first confrontation with hemorrhagic fevers. One of the consistent health problems in Panama was the deadly machupo virus, a member of the hemorrhagic fever group. Johnson joined a team to investigate machupo in Bolivia, where the disease was rampant. "We spent sixteen months in a village in the Bolivian rain forest. The town had 2,500 people. About 700 people got machupo in the time we were there and the fatality rate was about 18 percent.

"We were desperately hungry," remembers Johnson. "The food was terrible. Some of us began to eat the local white cheese. Others, who worried about getting brucella or TB from the dairy products, passed it up. Three of us came down with machupo. Luckily, we recovered, but that experience broke the biology of machupo. We learned that a particular kind of mouse was loaded with virus. I suspect that mouse urine got into the white cheese, although maybe the virus was spread as an aerosol. Once we determined the carrier of the virus, the Bolivians were very good about exterminating the mice. Now that town does not see more than ten cases of machupo a year."

The expertise gained in Bolivia was invaluable, but from his experiences Johnson knew enough about the hemorrhagic fevers to realize that the agent responsible, as in the cases of Legionnaire's disease and PCP, can be radically different.

Aware now of both the outbreak in Zaire and that in the Sudan, Johnson sought specimens that might identify the particular organism. That was not so easily arranged. With Belgian nationals involved, samples drawn from Sister Marie Jean's body had been flown to Antwerp for study. On learning of the affair in the Sudan, the British also got a man into Maridi from Nairobi. He collected specimens, which were sent to the British laboratory at Porton Down. Research on the two epidemics proceeded in two different countries.

"I don't want to accuse anyone of playing politics. There was a natural desire of the European labs to try to control the study, to get answers fast," says Johnson. "But neither Antwerp nor Porton Down had anywhere near the degree of experience that we had. The CDC was really the only outfit with the kind of trained medical sleuths, the methods and sufficient lab support to make a real investigation.

"Initially, people thought the disease might be yellow fever," continues Johnson. "WHO put a French expert on the scene, and he quickly cabled that this was no yellow fever epidemic because all of the mission staff at Yambuku had been vaccinated for that disease. From Geneva, WHO called the people at Antwerp, where they were blithely cooking along, inoculating things with stuff from the dead nun. WHO told Antwerp they were playing with fire, they didn't have the right containment facilities. Immediately, Antwerp shipped specimens to Porton Down, which was better equipped.

"When we found out that the people at Porton Down had everything, I got on the phone to a friend there, Ernie Bowen. He explained what they'd been doing. I told him that the tests they were using wouldn't work. We had a different system, using other materials. I offered to send him the stuff and asked if he would return the favor by letting us have a little bit of the specimens from Zaire. He said he couldn't. Everything was in their maximum-security lab. I said okay and still shipped him things by plane. Bowen called the following day to say he'd received our materials and that he let me have a little bit of one specimen plus some drops of sera from the Sudan.

"It was a holiday on Friday when we received the package from Porton Down. The staff was off, so we ourselves went into our Maximum Containment Lab and started the cultures. Either Monday or Tuesday when we looked through the electron microscope, we saw the worms. The Belgian experts believed that the organism was a rabdo virus. It vaguely resembled rabies but was not. We decided it was Marburg virus."

Some nine years earlier, pharmaceutical workers at Marburg in West Germany had received a shipment of green monkeys from Africa for experimental use. Seven of the workers died from a mysterious viral infection which became known as Marburg fever or green monkey disease. Subsequently, Marburg killed several Yugoslavians and an Australian tourist in Africa. Its source and means of spreading had never been discovered.

The diagnosis of a Marburg epidemic galvanized the CDC to organize an expedition to Africa bringing the only weapon believed effective against the disease; convalescent plasma drawn from survivors of Marburg fever. The CDC team was almost ready to embark when Dr. Patricia Webb, who had continued to test specimens, grabbed Johnson just as he left a rescue mission meeting with CDC Director Sencer. "It doesn't react," she reported, meaning that the fluorescent test for Marburg antibodies was negative. What looked like Marburg under the microscope was actually a different agent.

Even though they were no longer dealing with Marburg, Johnson and company still prepared to leave for Zaire. Meanwhile, the WHO French specialist already in Zaire had secured some new specimens. He had managed to find the now stricken wife of the first person believed to have developed the disease, and had drawn samples from her while she was on her deathbed. The small shipment, vials packed in cotton and wood, arrived at the CDC. Either because of fear or haste, the WHO operative had not centrifuged the specimens but simply had sent frozen whole blood.

"When we opened the package," recalls Johnson with a wry smile, "and read what it contained, we realized the criti-

cal specimen was the one from the dying wife. It happened
to be the only tube that had been smashed in transit. In the
lab, we wrung out the cotton packing with its dried blood
from the broken tube. We were able to get two or three drops.
They looked like coffee grounds, but they gave us a beautiful
reading, proving for sure the agent was something other than
Marburg."

The virus was eventually dubbed Ebola for a small river
in the vicinity of the Zairian epidemic.

Johnson and EIS officer Dr. Joel Breman took off for
Zaire's capital, Kinshasa. Political implications dogged the
effort. The Zairian government never fully accepted the notion of a WHO team to supersede its own minister of health,
so Johnson became head of a motley collection of American,
French, Belgian, and Canadian experts known as the International Medical Commission.

By the time the Americans arrived in Kinshasa, the nun who
had accompanied Marie Jean from Yambuku had also died
of Ebola. Worse, a native nurse who had attended Marie
Jean had now sickened. "She was already in terrible shape
when I saw her," says Johnson. "Unfortunately, before she
showed any symptoms, she had several days off and spent
them running all over Kinshasa. When she did become sick,
she tried three other hospitals. None would admit her. Only
on the fourth day of her illness did she go to ground at
Ngaliema. The drums were beating; the city was in an uproar
even though the government was trying to suppress the news
from Yambuku. People knew about the epidemic. In fact, all
of the European airlines that regularly fly to Johannesburg
ordinarily stopped at Kinshasa. They were on the point of
closing all European airports to any plane that stopped in
Kinshasa."

Johnson's immediate concern was to prevent widespread
contagion in Kinshasa. "Until we arrived there, no serious
precautions were taken. At Ngaliema, all they did was put the
sick in an isolated room. Nobody wore gowns, gloves, or
masks. I was very worried that somebody on our team would
get sick. We had no notion of how communicable the disease
was."

Infection through hospital contact was now being controlled, but the dying Zairian nurse had moved among the

general population of Kinshasa for four days. "We wanted to find all of the people with whom she had face-to-face contact," says Johnson, "which was a helluva job. Margaret Isaacson of South Africa had been invited to Zaire, because South Africa had some plasma for Marburg. Margaret organized a system to quarantine the entire hospital staff and anyone who had come in contact with the three victims. We located and the police incarcerated about fifty people. The government in Kinshasa was quite cooperative. They reacted a helluva lot different about the death of three people in the capital city as against 300 in the bush."

The 300 in the bush, however, became the focus of the International Medical Commission and the subject of Johnson's associate, EIS officer Dr. Joel Breman. Ordinarily, he was assigned to the Michigan Health Department. "I had lived in Africa in my youth," says Breman, "and I spoke French. That's why I was tapped."

Breman admits he was not prepared for how fast things were moving. "We arrived in the early morning and immediately attended a meeting of the commission under the minister of health. There must have been twenty people at the table and the minister said, 'This commission has done a lot of work. It has been arranged for a group to go to the epidemic area this morning.' Heads swung around and I realized they were looking at me. That was how I learned I was headed for Yambuku."

About twenty-four hours after he arrived in Kinshasa, Breman was debarking from a Zairian military plane at the rough strip serving Yambuku. "They pulled up the gangplank very fast. The crew were afraid of people trying to escape to Kinshasa. The Yambuku hospital had closed several days before we got there. Three of the nursing sisters, one of the fathers, and seven people who worked there had died. The remainder of the staff had run away. There was panic, fear. A quarantine barred anyone from the area. There were no cigarettes, no cooking oil or beer. No planes would land. Ships would not stop at the nearest port. There was a feeling of helplessness. The people felt they were being punished, somehow."

Oddly enough, Breman and his associates were reassured by the wildness of the tales by inhabitants. "We were told that everyone in a village had gotten the disease and that everyone had died. We knew that just couldn't be true. We set out to determine just how many people had become sick, what the fatalities actually were. We looked for active cases, trying to collect useful specimens."

The team carried with it a number of drugs, but they had little confidence in them. Bremen confesses to some anxious moments. "We took our temperatures three or four times a day to warn against the first hint of infection. I broke out in a rash, which made me nervous, but that proved to be just an allergy to sand flies."

Some time after Johnson and Breman were on their way to Africa, Dr. David Heymann, fresh from his duty in Philadelphia in pursuit in Legionnaire's disease, was aboard a plane headed for the National Aeronautical and Space Agency center in Houston. The CDC was determined to provide the best health care possible in the event any of the investigators caught Ebola. "Plans had been made to evacuate anyone who became sick," says Heymann, "but the airlines required us to have a means to isolate any person who was ill. For one dollar, NASA sold us a Vickers Isolator, a silver trailer they used when the astronauts came back from the moon. It loaded neatly into a C-130."

The apparatus was airlifted to Kinshasa and held in readiness for any members of the medical team who became infected. Heymann's talents were put to work in epidemiological surveys, and he eventually went to Yambuku to gather more evidence.

Meanwhile, the Kinshasa team wanted to open a second front against the Ebola epidemic in Sudan. But the effort called for someone already blooded in the ways of hemorrhagic viruses. There was a resource already in Africa, and its background is significant in the entire CDC effort.

About 1,500 miles from Kinshasa, in Sierra Leone, there was a Lassa fever station. Lassa, another hemorrhagic virus, had a major influence upon the CDC's operations. In 1969 the disease was discovered by the West when a virulent epidemic killed several American nurses who worked at a Church of the Brethren mission in Lassa, Nigeria.

Tropical-disease experts in the U.S. arranged for tissue samples from the infected nurses (two of whom had succumbed) to be scrutinized at a Yale University research laboratory. There, Dr. Jordi Casals studied the specimens under electron microscopes and experimented with mice, which did not live very long after being injected with sera from the human victims. Aware of the deadly potential of the Lassa organisms, Casals exercised great caution. Nevertheless, he fell desperately ill and only survived after receiving transfusions from a nurse who had recovered from an attack of Lassa fever.

Less fortunate was a Yale lab technician, Juan Roman. Although he had not even worked with the infected mice, somehow Roman sickened with Lassa while visiting relatives in Pennsylvania, where no one even knew that Lassa fever existed. Roman died, and Yale suspended its investigations into Lassa.

Because of what had happened at Yale, the CDC hastened to build a special facility for handling dangerous organisms —the Maximum Containment Laboratory. Karl Johnson was heavily involved in the planning. "I went to Fort Detrick [the U.S. Army center for research on biological weapons] and I stole their ideas on how to protect yourself in a lab. The safety officer there gave me some very good advice."

The CDC divides lab work into four categories. In Class I, people work at an open bench with vaccinia like polio. The staff have all been vaccinated; there's no danger of their becoming infected by the particular organisms. Class II is slightly more restricted; the people use a hood arrangement, instead of an open bench. In Class III with agents such as smallpox and Q fever, special laminar-flow hood rooms provide a self-contained air supply.

Class IV, high-containment, involves working with the most lethal specimens. Hemorrhagic viruses are among them. The Maximum Containment Laboratory is designed particularly for work with Class III and IV organisms. For direct handling of specimens, scientists enter through a gasketed, pressured door that seals tight. Anyone who enters must shower and change to sterilized clothing. On leaving, he must shower and change again. The floors are specially sealed; spills cannot seep into cracks in the floor or the walls. No walls are penetrated. All electrical wiring and plumbing lines lie outside the walls. Toilet materials do not enter the CDC sewage system until they have been held in storage tanks and specially treated.

The labs feature negative air pressure. In the unlikely event of a leak inside some component of the lab, the higher pressure of the external atmosphere contains everything inside the lab.

In sensitive areas, personnel wear suits resembling those of moon walkers with their own intake and exhaust systems. While the precautions eliminate the possibility that any Andromeda strain will escape to terrorize the public, the chief purpose of the Maximum Containment Lab is to protect the staff. So far the safety record is perfect, but people at the CDC still remember the two deaths in the rickettsial lab during the investigation of Legionnaires' disease.

The discovery of Lassa fever not only spurred the building of the special lab but also brought about the monitoring stations for the disease in Africa. Among the international crew staffing the Sierra Leone outpost was Dr. Joe Mc-Cormick.

"I was a teacher in Zaire as a member of the Peace Corps," says McCormick, whose Bachelor of Science degree was from Florida Southern. "When I wasn't at the school, I worked in the local hospital. That got me interested in medicine. I applied to medical school; a friend gave me the test in Zaire. Tropical diseases always interested me, and I spent my junior year at Harvard in tropical medicine."

McCormick, however, secured his residency in pediatrics before signing up with the EIS. When he completed his two-year term, McCormick continued on the CDC staff and was packed off to the Lassa fever research project.

Hearing of the new hemorrhagic fever epidemic, Mc-Cormick volunteered to join the international team. "I flew first to the Ivory Coast and caught a plane to Kinshasa, a distance of about 1,500 miles in about twenty-four hours." That may seem unexceptional to Western minds but it is extraordinarily quick in an area where one can wait from a day to a week for a "scheduled" flight. McCormick was immediately assigned to contact Breman at Yambuku.

There was a gnawing fear in Kinshasa for the safety of the squad in Yambuku. They had been scheduled to return after three days, but a week passed without any sign of them. Karl

Johnson was aware that the Zairian pilots were refusing to return to Yambuku, but that did not explain the lack of communications from Breman.

McCormick set about using his knowledge of the bush. He located an old radio transmitter in a mission on the outskirts of Kinshasa, about as close as one could get to signal Yambuku. Literate in Portuguese, Spanish, and French, McCormick exercised his linguistic skills to anyone listening in the Yambuku region. For hours he fiddled with the dials, searching the network of missions scattered throughout the isolated territory. Finally, in French, he contacted a Belgian who claimed to know the location of Breman and the others. Employing all of his diplomatic arts, McCormick persuaded the missionary to embark on a grueling two-hour trek in a Land Rover to the heart of the epidemic. The missionary found Breman, calmly going about his business, unaware of any anxiety over him, and drove him back to the mission station with the good news that the unit was safe and still awaiting transportation back to Kinshasa.

McCormick's work had only just begun. There was still an urgent need to look into the Sudanese epidemic and determine any linkage with the one in Zaire. The sites were separated by 800 unmapped miles. "We loaded eight men, two Land Rovers, food, medical supplies, and thirty barrels of diesel fuel into a C-130, and the Zairian air force flew us to a place midway between Yambuku and the Sudanese site of the heaviest infection." While one group headed off toward Yambuku, McCormick led his small band into the Sudan. The three-week, 1,000-mile trek took them through a thick rain forest, across the savannah past herds of elephants and hordes of antelopes, and over crocodile-filled rivers, the Land Rovers precariously perched on planks with leaky canoes nudging the cargoes across the rivers. The team interrogated and examined villagers, searching for signs of Ebola, clues to indicate the route of infection.

"We went from village to village, using the rough maps of the area. They showed the main roads, but they weren't terribly accurate, and it was a matter of looking for villages off the track. There were no trails; you'd walk through bush and grass. We'd ask if anyone who'd previously been well had suddenly come down with a high fever, bled from the mouth, or died suddenly. We would learn where the nearest clinic or hospital was, visit it, and find out if local health people had seen any cases."

At the Sudanese border, McCormick again relied upon his gift of gab to talk the team through bureaucratic resistance. Eventually, they penetrated 100 miles into Sudan over rutted, pitted dirt roads to the town of Nzara. There the scientists picked over the remnants of the Ebola outbreak who had survived the rampaging infection and collected specimens that proved the disease in the Sudan and Zaire was the same.

McCormick and company returned to Kinshasa, where Breman and his unit had brought their data. The International Medical Commission pieced together some pieces of the Ebola puzzle. "Although the hospital in Yambuku had closed, we found Sister Genieve," remembers Joel Breman. "She was a dynamic person who knew what had gone on. In late August, a 44-year-old man who had taught at the mission school came to the hospital because of a fever. They thought he had malaria and gave him chloroquine. Temporarily his fever dropped but then in four days it reached over 102°. In a week he was dead of severe hemorrhaging. The mission hospital at Yambuku issued five syringes and needles to the nursing staff each morning for use with all patients. Sometimes, between patients, they rinsed the equipment in a pan of warm water. At the end of the day sometimes, equipment was boiled for sterilization." With 6,000 to 12,000 outpatients a month at the hospital, and such obviously unsanitary procedures, the opportunities for an epidemic were all in place when the unfortunate teacher carrying the Ebola organism received his chloroquine by hypodermic.

The investigators found that almost all of the first cases were transmitted by contaminated hypodermics. Later the disease spread from person-to-person contact, as no effort was made to isolate the sick people and they returned to their villages and homes. The toll over the seven weeks of the epidemic was 318 cases; 218 died.

Findings in the Sudan were remarkably similar. There too, the flash point of the epidemic centered on the local hospital.

The IMC disbanded, leaving a number of unanswered questions. Although McCormick and the others collected specimens of wildlife, small mammals and insects, the reservoir for Ebola continued a mystery. No clues to how the first case at Yambuku became infected were found. No link between the Sudan and the Zaire infections was discovered. However, while the borders are controlled, freebooters constantly smuggle contraband through the area. That might account for the almost simultaneous outbreaks 800 miles apart.

About ten months later, word reached Johnson that a girl had died of acute hemorrhagic illness in Tandala, a village some 200 miles from Yambuku. Learning the victim never had been in contact with anyone from the previous epidemic, Johnson and CDC people in the Maximum Containment Lab isolated Ebola in her blood. Further research turned up an American missionary in the area, Dr. Thomas Cairns, who worked at the Tandala Mission Hospital. His blood tests showed Ebola antibodies.

Cairns recalled having cut his finger in 1972 while performing an autopsy on a patient who died of what was diagnosed then as yellow fever. Convinced that the dead man had Ebola, Johnson theorized that the disease must have a natural reservoir in the Zaire River Basin.

He had to wait eighteen months before he could test his hypothesis. There were no funds for a search of the Zaire River Basin environment. Serendipity finally offered a trip. Because of fears of a monkey pox epidemic (the disease is a close kin to smallpox), WHO organized a control party to the region and Johnson got himself invited with the understanding that he might also collect specimens that might explain Ebola.

"We went to Yosalemba, about 80 miles to the west of Yambuku. There had been some Ebola cases there, and the place had exactly the same ecology as Tambala and Yambuku. It was rain forest with an unbelievable variety of life, quite like what I had seen in Bolivia. We figured the best possibility was mammals and we took about 1,500 specimens. We brought the materials back to Atlanta. It was all negative, very disappointing," admits Johnson, who had been sure he would find the answer.

Stumped, the CDC experts waited with mixed emotions for another opportunity to study Ebola. The scourge boiled up

in September 1979 at Nzara in Sudan. "On a Friday afternoon
in Atlanta," remembers Dr. Roy Baron, a handsome, clean-
shaven young physician, "I was having lunch in the cafeteria
when my supervisor came up to me and with a big grin asked,
'Do you want to go to the Sudan?' I smiled back and said
sure. We'd heard there was again Ebola activity in the Sudan.
I was told to see Joe McCormick and that we would probably leave on Monday."

Baron had just completed his EIS tour and had been accepted on the staff of the unit concerned with, among other
things, tropical disease. "Instead of getting ready for two
more days," remembers Baron, "we flew out the following
morning. In Geneva, the people at WHO briefed us. I spent
my time going over crates of equipment, diagnostic instruments, disposable caps, gowns, gloves. We flew overnight to
Khartoum, where we were supposed to make a connection
to Juba, the southern capital.

"Joe and I split up temporarily. I stayed in Khartoum waiting for them to unload the gear while he caught the last flight
to Juba. For five days I tried to get a plane. The government
offered a Piper Cub, which would have held me and one of
my thirteen crates. Finally, the Sudanese military took me to
Juba, but Joe and I were stuck there for days trying to get
transportation to Nzara. We needed a good-size airplane for
our stuff; none was available. Somebody said the chief of
police would fly us down, but he wanted to take his wife and
girl friend, which left no room for the stuff we needed. It was
bizarre, the way private interest and public responsibility
conflicted in some places." Finally the team located a Beech-
craft big enough to ferry them and their equipment. The
scene in Nzara shocked Baron. "It was an eerie scene in the
dispensaries," says he. "You walked into a single large room
with a thatched roof. The attendants were like ghosts in white
robes with lanterns. It was quite tragic. The bedpans beside
the beds were filled with blood; the dying lay there very
stoic. We went from patient to patient, eight to ten in a room.
We spent the first days with the examining people until 10:00
or 11:00 at night. We took specimens, found a hand centri-
fuge, spun-cranked it with all our might, then froze the
plasma specimens and put them aboard planes out of Nzara."

Both men prowled the area hunting suspected cases. "We

heard of fifty-seven," says McCormick, "and we tracked down every one of them. There was a German nurse with me, and we spent one entire day walking through grass taller than us looking for three cases. The people were cooperative but they were distressed about what would happen to someone taken to the hospital."

Routine precautions required strict isolation of anyone who might harbor Ebola. Family members could not visit the sick. In the event of a death, clothing was destroyed and burials were immediate, without the traditional washing of the body and the ceremonial touching, dressing, and vigils.

"The local people occasionally tried to haul away the bodies of the dead," says McCormick, "because they assumed they wouldn't be permitted to perform a proper funeral."

Protocol called for Baron and McCormick to shield themselves with portable respirators squirted with formaldahyde, disposable paper gowns, and gloves. But the heat was staggeringly oppressive, particularly with a respirator on, and Baron and McCormick occasionally discarded their respirators and risked infection in order to proceed. In the field one day, disaster struck. "Joe was taking a blood specimen from a potential victim," recalls Baron. "The woman flinched as Joe tried to draw blood, and the needle stuck Joe in his finger. We rationalized that because Joe didn't bleed, he was okay. We knew from experience, however, that anyone infected by a needle puncture invariably developed a fatal case. The only treatment we had was some serum taken from a former Ebola patient. The antibodies were supposed to help.

"I was very worried, but Joe seemed unconcerned. We met some people for dinner and we stayed up drinking until 3:00 a.m. I kept trying to get Joe out of there so I could give him some serum, but he was really wound up and just kept talking. Finally, I managed to get him away and gave him two units of the serum.

"A few days later we learned that the woman involved in the accident did not have Ebola. It was fortunate, because when we tested McCormick for antibodies, he had none. The serum we received was also not from someone who had recovered from Ebola."

In Nzara, enforcement of strict measures to prevent the spread of infection helped considerably. The epidemic killed twenty-two of the fifty-seven identified cases but burned out quickly in contrast to the Yambuku and Maridi outbreaks.

McCormick discovered that the first victim in Nzara had worked in a local cotton mill. Still, the examination of rats, bats, and insects that inhabited the place revealed no traces of an Ebola source. It was another blind alley.

The forces of modern medicine again withdrew, still baffled. Then in 1980, Karl Johnson in Atlanta received a telephone call from Dr. Thomas Cairns, the medical missionary from Tambala whose experience with Ebola had sent Johnson off on his fruitless hunt to the Zaire River Basin.

Two kids from a family raising guinea pigs near Tandala had entered the mission hospital, where they died of hemorrhagic symptoms. Cairns was submitting samples of their blood along with specimens from the family's crop of guinea pigs, a number of which had died just before the children became sick. The CDC lab, however, diagnosed hepatitis and sickle-cell anemia as the causes of the two boys' deaths. Johnson turned his attention to other avenues of research.

About three months later, he received a second call from Cairns. "I'm at Kennedy Airport," said Cairns.

"What are you doing here?" Johnson asked.

"You remember how I got infected with Ebola doing an autopsy?" said Cairns. "Well, I've done it again. This time it was a woman with fulminating hepatitis. When I was performing the autopsy, I cut myself. I think it's a very bad strain of hepatitis."

"I invited him to come to Atlanta for gamma globulin, which they did not have in Africa," remembers Johnson, who grins at recalling the conversation. "He told me he had already booked himself on a flight to Atlanta.

"After he came and we gave him the gamma globulin, we talked and reviewed our recent studies. We decided to retest the samples we had from the two boys. Nobody realized that mixed in with those specimens were samples drawn from the guinea pigs. Antibodies to human infections of Ebola showed up in a fluorescent test. Checking, we realized the guinea pig specimens mixed with the samples from the boys had been infected with Ebola. We got excited, and Sally Stansfield from the CDC went to Tandala and collected 140 guinea pigs and insects from around the houses. We tested them and found that 20 percent of the guinea pigs had antibodies to Ebola. But as far as finding the virus itself [rather than antibodies], we came up with a blooming zip." The virus itself had mysteriously vanished, leaving behind, like a footprint to prove it had been there, its antibodies.

In the years since the CDC first became aware of the hemorrhagic viruses there has been considerable progress. Not only was a reservoir for machupo discovered in Bolivia, but also in Sierra Leone a CDC team headed by virologist Thomas Monath (and which included David Fraser before he directed the Legionnaires' disease team) detected the Lassa virus in the blood of a particular kind of rat. Eradication of this type of rat can control Lassa epidemics. Both machupo and Lassa fever victims benefit from plasma drawn from the blood of recovered victims of the diseases.

"There isn't any treatment for Ebola or Marburg. Plasma doesn't really do any good," says Johnson. "The biology of these diseases is different from Lassa and machupo. Even if the serum given Joe McCormick when he stabbed himself with a needle contained antibodies for Ebola, it would not have helped.

"We're still struggling with the problem," admits Johnson. He is no longer with the CDC, having transferred to the U.S. Army Medical Research Institute (USAMRI) at Fort Detrick. There he busies himself with the need to find a vaccine and then a treatment. The military's interest stems from the possibility that American forces may someday be sent to climes where these diseases exist or that they might somehow be made into weapons of biological warfare.

Joe McCormick now tends the CDC shop looking into the exotic viruses. He is only partially resigned to a desk job, with forays into the Maximum Containment Lab. "I've got years of field experience, but my responsibilities make it difficult to get away. Still, I enjoy getting out. . . ." And McCormick trails off in a kind of reverie, perhaps recalling his African days.

David Heymann spends his time on investigations of malaria, while Joel Breman is engaged in smallpox research. Roy Baron is puzzling over one of the knottiest problems to bedevil the CDC, the mysterious deaths of thirty-nine refugees from Laos, Hmongs, young men in their 20s and 30s who suddenly expired at night in their beds without any warning. Intensive studies by pathologists have failed to reveal the reasons their healthy hearts stopped.

Ebola's answer is even more tantalizing. The guinea pigs of Tandala are not the reservoirs of the disease any more than the green monkeys are responsible for Marburg. In both instances, since the animals themselves fall victim they cannot be considered the carriers. "The guinea pigs may serve as a kind of sentinel," says McCormick.

The ghastly specter of an invasion by hemorrhagic virus hangs over the United States. Several people who contracted Lassa fever in Africa have arrived in the States with the disease. Fortunately, person-to-person contagion so far is not the major means by which the hemorrhagic viruses spread. Also, the known reservoirs of hemorrhagic viruses, a particular strain of mice and the African rat of Lassa fever, have shown, as yet, no ability to survive outside their natural habitat. But it is a well-known and chilling fact that some viruses have a way of mutating and making themselves adaptable to environments. Until the sources of Ebola and Marburg are known, these viruses cannot be entirely eliminated as a threat to the U.S. The Maximum Containment Lab and scientists like Joe McCormick must continue research and vigilance against the awful possibility that hemorrhagic fevers will invade this country.

CHAPTER
11

The Black Death in New Mexico

JOHN BIGBEE (pseudonym), a 28-year-old Navajo who lived in a trailer in the hamlet of Cuba, New Mexico, awoke on the morning of May 29, 1981, with achy muscles, a sore throat, and pains in his head. Over the next few days, his symptoms worsened, and he sought treatment from several different Indian medicine men. The rituals performed by the shamans did not seem to help, and Bigbee finally showed up at the Cuba Health Center. Examined by a physician's assistant, Bigbee continued to complain of his original symptoms, and his temperature registered 101°F. His nasal passages appeared inflamed, his tonsils oozed, and the back of his neck felt sore. The diagnosis was streptococcal pharyngitis, a bacterial infection originating in his nose. Bigbee received doses of penicillin and aspirin and returned to his home.

The symptoms abated in a day or so, but then John Bigbee felt worse than ever, although his complaints had changed. Now he had difficulty breathing; when he coughed, Bigbee brought up flecks of blood. Accompanied by his mother and a sister, Bigbee was driven by his brother to consult a medicine man in northwestern New Mexico, a considerable distance from Cuba. The particular shaman Bigbee sought, however, was not to be found. With the sick man in much greater distress, his family then drove him to the emergency suite at the Gallup Indian Medical Center.

"He was breathing very rapidly," says Dr. Molly Ettenger, the physician who attended Bigbee in Gallup. "He looked about as sick as anyone could. He kept bringing up sputum tinged with blood." Wheezing, gasping for air, Bigbee was rushed from emergency to an upstairs intensive-care ward. "He was able to talk but not for any length because he was having such trouble with his respiration," recalls Ettenger. "He kept saying, 'I can't breathe,' and we started asking questions to find out what he might have. He insisted that he hadn't been around any animals from whom he might have picked up something that could affect his lungs. He also said he didn't drink. Frequently when you see young men with this kind of pneumonia condition, they're alcoholics. The family members who were with him told us that he didn't drink, and to the best of their knowledge he hadn't been around any animals recently."

Bigbee did not volunteer information about his search for an Indian medicine man; the investigators only learned of his resort to this kind of cure later. "Sometimes we see people who are covered with ashes after a medicine man's ceremony," says Ettenger, "but Bigbee did not have any signs of ashes. He did have some small bruises, but they were smaller than what I've seen on a person treated by a medicine man. The man just deteriorated rapidly in front of our eyes," continues Ettenger. "We already were going to intubate him [put him on an artificial respirator] when he went into cardiac arrest. A nurse did mouth-to-mouth resuscitation until we could get him on the respirator. But he lost consciousness. We kept his heart beating through life-support apparatus for a few hours, but it was hopeless and he died."

Even as the staff at the Gallup hospital futilely labored to save Bigbee from his unknown ailment, the technicians in the lab were running tests on samples of his tissue. "They had a sample of what he coughed up under a microscope," says Ettenger. "The bacteria were very strange to me, the biggest and fattest organisms I'd ever seen. Also there were so many of them."

The Gallup lab scientists thought they recognized the bacteria as *Yersinia pestis*—bubonic plague, the black death—but curiously enough when they attempted a test that would trigger an antibody reaction for plague, it was negative. Nevertheless, the word was flashed to the state health department that a patient appeared to have died of pneumonic plague.

Accounts of bubonic plague during the days of the Roman Empire are grim: "The houses were filled with dead bodies and the streets with funerals; neither age nor sex was exempt; slaves and plebeians were suddenly taken off amidst the lamentations of their wives and children, who, while they assisted the sick and mourned the dead, were seized with the disease, and perishing, were burned on the same funeral pyre." If anything, the reputation of the scourge grew more horrible starting in the fourteenth century. Plague cut its way through the Far East before moving into Europe through Italy; the Genovese are believed to have transported plague in their cargoes of silks and spices, as they transported cholera. In the first attacks during the fourteenth century, three-quarters of the citizens of Siena died; almost the same proportion perished at Pisa. Poet Petrarch observed the epidemic in Florence: "We go out of doors, walk through street after street and find them full of dead and dying, and when we get home again we find no live thing within the house, all having perished in the brief interval of our absence."

Boccaccio, Petrarch's contemporary, offered a graphic description of the disease. "There appeared certain tumors in the groin, or under the armpits, some as big as a small apple others as an egg; and afterward purple spots in most parts of the body." The author of the *Decameron* was describing lymph-gland swellings, which were called buboes; hence "bubonic" plague. The dark discolorations also were responsible for the name black death, which the disease earned when it overwhelmed England, wreaking such havoc that the dead were piled in trenches while members of Parliament and all other people of means fled the cities. Almost half of Europe died from the black death between the fourteenth and seventeenth centuries. Some blamed the curse upon the Jews, others argued an offense to an angry God. The sect of the flagellants revived; they whipped themselves to placate the Almighty. Others decided that since infection and death were inevitable, pure hedonism was the only supportable way of life. In Europe, the disease suddenly died out after 300 years. The decline has been attributed by some scholars to the invasion of the brown rat from Central Asia. Great hordes of them were seen swimming the Volga River during the eighteenth century as they migrated west. They quickly displaced *Rattus rattus* as the dominant rodent. That was significant, because the source of the bacterium responsible for bubonic plague is a flea with an affinity for rodents. However, unlike *Rattus rattus*, the brown rat was not attracted to human habitation. In addition, its particular flea did not consider humans as tasty as did the fleas associated with *Rattus rattus*. The people of Britain were also cleansed of plague by an apparent disaster. The great London fire burned much of the city, consuming in the flames, along with buildings and people, the bearers of plague.

When plague reappeared toward the end of the nineteenth century in Hong Kong, medical science was far enough advanced to have noticed a connection with rats. Working independently, the Swiss scientist Alexander Yersin (a pupil of Louis Pasteur) and the Japanese Shibasaburo Kitasato (a student of Robert Koch, who, among other deeds, isolated cholera's cause) discovered the bacillus responsible for plague. Yersin dubbed it *Pasturella pestis* in honor of his mentor, but some years ago the World Health Organization felt the discoverer deserved the recognition, and now plague's short thick bacterial rod is officially *Yersinia pestis*.

Originally, the organism was associated with the Asian black rat, but scientists then realized the actual carrier is a flea which bears *Yersinia pestis* in its blood. The infection results from the bite of the flea. Many kinds of rodents and mammals may harbor the flea.

The United States witnessed brief outbreaks of plague during colonial times; the most recent severe epidemic occurred in San Francisco in 1907 when 167 people reportedly perished.

Since then, plague has been only a sporadic threat in the States, confined to the Southwest but occasionally cropping up elsewhere—Denver saw a nasty outbreak several years ago, and another occurred in the Pacific Northwest. "As an EIS officer," recalls Don Francis, "I had literally just driven to Oregon in my van with my family when I was sent off to Pendleton [Oregon] because of a case of bubonic plague."

For all its deadly history, plague is ordinarily not a highly epidemic disease in the U.S., because in its most common manifestation, contagion is strictly through rodent-loving fleas. The excellent sanitation and rodent control in American cities restricts the rodent population and their plague-bearing fleas. The fleas turn to humans only in the absence of a more desirable host such as rats, prairie dogs, and squirrels. When Albert Camus wrote his great novel *The Plague* against the backdrop of a North African epidemic, the action begins with the rats coming out of the sewers to die in the streets. The local citizens are puzzled but unconcerned, not realizing that having destroyed their sources of life, the fleas will be forced to turn to the next available hosts, humans.

Plague is usually an insect-borne infection, but there is a notable exception. Once a human is infected, the bacillus can make its way to the lungs, to become pneumonic plague. In such instances the sick person becomes a potential infector of everyone with whom he comes into contact, breathing, coughing, and sneezing the bacteria into the air. Fortunately for others, individuals with the plague usually either die or recover before the infection reaches their lungs. During the great epidemics of the Middle Ages, presumably the infections passed from human to human, because a number of cases of the pneumonic form of the disease occurred. Because plague can be spread through the air it has been an attractive candidate for those developing biological-warfare weapons.

On the afternoon of June 5, at the New Mexico State Scientific Laboratory, Linda Nims performed a fluorescent antibody test on a sample of tissue from the body of John Bigbee. Although, like her Gallup counterparts, Nims had difficulty producing the expected plague antibody reaction, she was certain still that Gallup had a case of plague. At 5:30 p.m. that Friday, she telephoned the Plague Branch, Vector-Borne Viral Diseases Division of the CDC in Fort Collins, Colorado. This outpost of the CDC has the mission to track infections spread by insects. Among the Fort Collins responsibilities are tularemia (rabbit fever), Rocky Mountain spotted fever—a tick-borne ailment of which there is far more east of the Mississippi than in the regions from which it draws its name—and bubonic plague. When a specimen from Bigbee was shipped to Fort Collins for inspection, the lab scientists created a subculture of the organisms, diluting them sufficiently for a confirmed antibody reaction.

Unfortunately, John Bigbee was one of those rare cases of pneumonic plague. The disease was in his lungs. He could easily have infected dozens of people, including the staff at the hospital. Although the antibiotics tetracycline and chloramphenicol, sometimes in conjunction with streptomycin, are highly effective in treating plague, the disease can still be fatal if not treated early enough. Anyone with whom Bigbee had contact was in danger of losing his or her life.

On Saturday morning, June 6, a pair of CDC investigators, physician Robert B. Craven and zoologist Gary Maupin, flew from Fort Collins to Albuquerque, rented a car, and drove 75 miles to Torreon.

Gary Maupin's credentials included an M.S. in zoology and a minor concentration in entymology. He had been with the CDC's Plague Branch for eleven years, and when not in the field he worked in the lab testing mammals and fleas for signs of *Yersinia pestis*. Robert Craven studied medicine at the University of Virginia and received an EIS appointment in 1972. "I was originally working in viral diseases," says Craven, "but I've worked more on plague than anything else."

The first stop for the pair of investigators was the Bigbee home on the Navajo reservation in Torreon. Craven remembers, "There were maybe four rooms for about six people and the walls were constructed of wire with a kind of stucco plastered over them. They had running water in the house, but the toilets were all outdoors. There were also sheds for grain storage and rabbit pens plus a lot of refuse strewn over the ground. It all provided plenty of what we call rodent harborage. The family also told us everything they knew of Bigbee's movements and habits, with whom he associated." The observations made by the team and the information from the family suggested several routes of action. The home and its environs would be searched for fleas that might be infected, and the investigators had the names of people whom Bibgee might have infected.

From the family and from later interviews with Molly Ettenger, the health authorities also pieced together the ghastly saga of Bigbee's final day of life. Bigbee felt considerably worse on the morning of June 4, and rather than return to the Cuba Health Center, which had apparently failed to cure him, he decided to seek help from a particular shaman in the town of Shiprock, to the north and west of the family home on the reservation lands about Torreon. Bigbee, his mother, one sister, and a brother, who did the driving, drove through the arid, hot hills and valleys of the state on a course that looped up into southern Colorado before dipping down to the destination in New Mexico. Unfortunately, the medicine man whom Bigbee sought was unavailable.

His condition had continued to deteriorate during the long trek. It was apparent to all that he required treatment. Unfortunately, although there was an Indian medical center in Shiprock, the family decided to head for Gallup, still another two hours away. As Molly Ettenger learned from the supervisors later, "He was continually coughing and wheezing during the trip, spraying his family with countless organisms within the confines of the car." Indeed, in the emergency room at Gallup and subsequently during the final desperate efforts to save him, Bigbee vented clouds of sputum drenched in plague bacillus.

Craven and Maupin contacted officials in the Indian Health Service and the state public health agencies to alert them to the potential of an epidemic of pneumonic plague. Personnel from these organizations embarked on a hunt for every person who had come near Bigbee during the final days of his life. For example, the medicine men on the reservations were visited and tested for signs of plague. Family members, neighbors, casual acquaintances, and, of course, the staff at both the Cuba Health Center and at Gallup, particularly those who treated Bigbee, were examined for any signs of plague.

"It was fairly easy at the hospital," says Robert Craven, "to find who had contact with Bigbee and then watch them for any signs of infection."

In the cases of some individuals, however, the threat was so great that direct preventive medicine was indicated. When Bigbee suffered cardiac arrest while being prepped for an artificial respirator, a nurse had tried to sustain him with mouth-to-mouth resuscitation. To destroy any germs in her system, she received injections of tetracycline and streptomycin. Others at the hospital, including the anesthesiologist who had risked infection when he did the tracheotomy to insert a breathing tube in Bigbee's throat, went on a similar regimen. The family members who had accompanied Bigbee were given antibiotics also.

A vaccine for bubonic plague exists, and it confers limited immunity to the disease. CDC investigators usually do not rely on this kind of protection, however, for their periodic skirmishes with the disease. Instead, when their exposure warrants it, they receive tetracycline and streptomycin shots during the period of vulnerability to the disease. Maupin, for example, has been on the receiving end of such preventive therapy no less than seven times. However, in Cuba neither he nor Craven ever dealt directly with patients or infected animals. They merely kept a prudent watch on their health, prepared for treatment at the first signs of any symptoms. They were put on a standard prophylaxis antibiotic schedule to kill any nascent infections.

Tracking down the other people whom Bigbee had seen during the period when his infection might be contagious was another matter. "Since he was dead, we had to rely on the information given to us by his family, reconstructing what he had been doing," remarks Craven, "but they were very helpful."

The CDC representatives were extremely sensitive about their intrusion into the Indian culture. They worked in cooperation with the staff of the Indian health organizations and let professionals from those groups meet with the shamans and interrogate individuals on reservations. A total of seventy-four persons were identified as having been involved sufficiently with Bigbee to be at risk for plague. They included a woman practitioner of Indian medicine. Fifty-three people were designated for the preventive treatment and surveillance. Neither Bigbee's mother nor seven children in the family ever evinced any signs of the disease in their lung X-rays. The prompt surveillance and use of the preventive drugs appeared to have halted any development of an epidemic of pneumonic plague.

Meanwhile, Craven and Maupin concentrated upon discovering the extent of the plague infestation. "We were going to have to make major manpower recommendations for control of the epidemic, and we needed to know as much as possible about the length and breadth of the problem," says Craven. The pair focused upon Cuba and Torreon, looking for the pathways of contagion that had resulted in Bigbee's death. Maupin scouted the towns for the purpose of trapping animals and catching fleas.

"Cuba," says Maupin, "sits in a valley, made by the Puerco River. It's aptly named Pig River. It's very muddy, runs through the town. The Jemez Mountains are right behind the place. It's an old town lacking good sanitation, and the 2,000 people are spread out over about two square miles." In point of fact, neither investigator was that surprised at the involvement of Cuba. Less than three months before, a woman from the town had been diagnosed as a plague case. She recovered; there was a superficial attempt to wipe out infected animals, but CDC officials were not called to the scene.

"We saw very few prairie dogs or rock squirrels, which right away was suspicious," continues Maupin. "Ordinarily there would be plenty of rodent life around, starting at the treeline on the slopes of the Jemez range. The mill area, though, was completely antiseptic. You couldn't find any rodents within 300 yards around the place; the bark and sawdust was so sterile nothing could live in the waste from the mill.

"Bigbee had worked as a tree debarker at the sawmill," says Craven. "Those who knew him described Bigbee as quiet; spending his time between work either at his residence in Cuba or at the family home at Torreon 35 miles away. He did not hunt, which eliminated the possibility that he had come across *Yersinia pestis* in the wild." In the U.S. hunters have sometimes run afoul of *Yersinia pestis*. Indeed, CDC records contain a tale of two Air Force officers chasing rabbits in the brush. They nearly died from the plague carried by fleas aboard the cottontails they bagged. Less lucky was an Oregonian who contracted a fatal case of the disease from his kill after he skinned it.

To the best knowledge of Bigbee's family and friends, the homes in Torreon and Cuba were not infested with rodents, although there was some talk that rats had been seen in the vicinity of the sawmill. The investigators also learned that Bigbee was fond of a cat, several dogs in Torreon, and a neighbor's hound in Cuba.

"One long-shot theory," says Maupin, "was that Bigbee became infected while at his job. There's a glass housing to protect a worker from chips from a tree when the machine strips the bark. The glass cover, though, is not airtight. A dead squirrel with fleas could have been in one of the pieces of wood Bigbee debarked and the machinery could have manufactured an aerosol spray from the remains." While it is more likely that Bigbee became infected from his contact with domestic animals or by inadvertently coming too close to an infected prairie dog, the possibility suggested by Maupin indicates how difficult it is to protect people against plague.

From conversations with acquaintances, Craven learned that the cat with whom Bigbee had been on friendly terms had died in a car upon which the dead man had been working. That was a most promising lead. "It's been found," remarks Craven, "that cats can pass along plague bacillus through their saliva or by scratching a person. Actually, a vet working with a cat was bitten and he did develop the disease." The lead on the dead feline petered out when it was learned that the animal had died at least a month before Bigbee became ill; plague's incubation period is from two to six days ordinarily.

Although bubonic plague conjures up fearsome images, the people did not panic when news of the threat reached the media. For the general public the advice was to avoid contact with animals and to restrict outdoor activities by children. "The younger people knew what was going on," says Maupin. "As part of the health education program in the public and parochial schools they hear about such things. One man I talked to was thankful when we came around to his area for the rodent-elimination program. His three kids were out of school and had been stuck in the house. They were driving him up the wall.

"Several of the neighborhood dogs fondled by Bigbee tested out positive for plague antibodies, indicating *Yersinia pestis* had reached their bloodstream. They were not bearing any fleas, but while canines do not become seriously ill from plague, they can transmit the disease through their saliva or by biting a human while bearing an active infection," says Maupin. "In Ruidoso [New Mexico], a woman came down with plague from her pet dogs whom she allowed to sleep on her bed. They had carried the fleas into the house after chasing prairie dogs in the backyard."

Maupin set out his traps around the sawmill and trailer home in Cuba. The snares failed to catch any rodents, because the rodent population had all but disappeared. Around Torreon the hunters were more successful, bagging a number of squirrels, mice, and chipmunks. None of the specimens bore fleas harboring *Yersinia pestis*, nor did fluorescent antibody tests come up with any positives. For the animals, the plague apparently was so virulent the mortality rate was close to 100 percent—none survived long enough to manufacture antibodies or support infected fleas. Maupin then went on a flea hunt in the deserted prairie-dog burrows around Cuba. His paraphernalia consisted of a plumber's snake with an alligator clamp attached to one end. The clamp gripped a fuzzy white flannel diaper. "I would insert it as much as 6 feet into a burrow," says Maupin. "Any fleas looking for a host will stick to the diaper, and when you remove the snake from the burrow you can see the fleas quite clearly on the diaper. We anesthetize them with ether, pick them off, and drop them in a plastic bag marked for the location, and then take them to a 'plague mobile.' It's actually just a camper fitted out for field work." During these expeditions, Maupin received three flea bites, but he was able to examine his assailants, find no signs of *Yersinia pestis*, and therefore avoid a series of injections.

Altogether, Maupin, with Craven at his side, captured 964 fleas in Cuba, many of them riddled with *Yersinia pestis*. The New Mexico State Environmental Improvement Division immediately began a vigorous flea-eradication program, dusting the nesting sites and burrows of critters hospitable to fleas with carbaryl, a rodenticide. The per-burrow numbers of insects fell drastically within a month. However investigators still found some live ones packed with *Yersinia pestis*.

"It's unlikely that we can ever entirely eliminate plague," admits Craven, in spite of the sustained campaigns against the disease by the CDC and its local allies. "It seems to have the capacity to survive even the fiercest epizootic [an epidemic among animals]. The fleas just move to another kind of rodent. The best we can accomplish with any rodenticide program is to protect populated areas." The animals and their deadly guests cannot be totally destroyed in the wild.

The investigators from the CDC were convinced that

Yersinia pestis, which had ravaged the prairie dogs, inevitably came in contact with Bigbee and the woman victim earlier in the spring. (It's conceivable other people became sick but plague can run a mild course, and Indians on reservations or living isolated in the hills have been known to survive without being treated with Western medicine.)

The problem in Sandoval County was compounded by the people's ignorance of or unwillingness to be concerned by the presence around their homes of large numbers of rodents. Solid-waste disposal in the community has never been properly handled, and there is a tradition of *laissez faire* with garbage.

Obviously, there was a large die-off of the prairie dogs, a signal that the disease was rampant. "We asked people about this," says Craven, "and when we brought it to their attention, they said, 'Oh yeah, now that you mention it, we didn't see the prairie dogs around.'" The failure of people to react to the absence of usual numbers of prairie dogs may have cost John Bigbee his life.

The investigators had to ask themselves whether it was possible that when he first showed up at the Cuba Health Center, Bigbee should have been diagnosed as infected with plague. But the disease is so rare that even though there had been a case only two months before in Cuba, doctors in the clinic there tended not to think in terms of plague.

Molly Ettenger remembers seeing another plague victim a few months after Bigbee died. "This was a Gallup woman; she never even made it out of the emergency room. She died there," says Ettenger. But a year later, a young woman presented herself at Gallup and announced that she had bubonic plague. "She was right," says Ettenger, "although a few days before she had come to the hospital and been diagnosed with something else. The problem was that we hadn't seen any plague for several years so nobody considered it; it was that rare. Now, when someone comes in with a routine cold, there's a tendency to think, could it be plague?"

This is not to say that Bigbee actually had plague on his visit to the Cuba Health Center. "The evidence is that Bigbee did not have plague at the time," explains Craven. "It's unlikely that the antibiotics given to him would have eliminated his symptoms. Furthermore, when we examined several of his kin they had that same type of pharyngeal infection—

strep condition—Bigbee had. He probably had two separate illnesses; the problem was that the second time around, after he somehow came in contact with an infected flea, there was some delay before he was seen by a physician."

The success in wiping out pestilential forces was a temporary one. By the spring of 1982, an epizootic stretched across Navajo lands from New Mexico well into Arizona, with several new human plague victims. "We've had two mild winters with warm wet springs," says Maupin. "The animals have not gone into hibernation and have been more active, which means that the flea population has thrived."

The black death is alive and well in the U.S.

12

Getting into Heavy Metal

FRANKLIN, KENTUCKY, the seat of Simpson County, is in a rural section of the state and for the most part is dominated by tobacco farming. However, when several factories sprang up in Franklin, many of the local women were delighted to sign on. Among the new industries was Potter & Brumfield, which manufactured electromagnetic relays. Factory work at Potter & Brumfield was agreeable to the women. It meant year-round employment and an escape from the arduous task of harvesting the bottom leaves of tobacco plants and crawling around the fields on hands and knees.

Early in October 1965, Ethel Mae Turner (pseudonym), whose job consisted of wrapping copper wire around spindles in the coil room of Potter & Brumfield, felt her energy flagging, her spirits drooping. Turner had developed a pain at the back of her head which radiated down through the nape of her neck. Along with the aches came a light-headedness that affected Turner even more when she tried to walk. Not only was she physically woozy but she also began to slur her words. Her husband thought she was acting drunk. Since Ethel Mae was a confirmed teetotaler, her husband took her to see a local physician, Dr. Carter Moore.

Ethel Mae Turner's condition alarmed Dr. Moore, because several other women during the previous few days had stopped by with similar complaints, and he could not arrive at a diagnosis. One puzzling aspect was the absence of any significant fever, the usual sign of a bacterial or viral infection, either of which could explain the strange pains and neuromuscular reactions. As he had done with the handful of others manifesting the syndrome, Dr. Moore arranged to have Ethel Mae Turner admitted to the hospital.

Other physicians in Simpson County, including Dr. Thomas Kirby of Bowling Green, were also stumped by patients with these inexplicable difficulties. The nonplussed Kirby wrote beside each patient's name on his medical charts the word "poisoning."

All of the patients Carter Moore had seen were employees of Potter & Brumfield. The physician telephoned William Eldred, the factory manager, hoping an explanation might lie in some incident at the plant. Eldred assured Moore that he knew of no events at the factory that might be responsible. However, with notable prudence, Eldred immediately notified the parent company, AMC Corp. The insurance company responsible for workman's compensation now sought information. Dr. Moore had also alerted the state epidemiologist, Dr. Joseph Skaggs, a veterinarian. He arranged for a pair of industrial hygienists to visit the factory and look for an explanation.

None of these investigations produced any answers, and Kirby took it upon himself to telephone the CDC for guidance. The case load now totaled twenty-five. The CDC requested an invitation from the state health department, and subsequently, EIS officer Dr. George Miller flew from Atlanta to the Kentucky site.

Kirby suggested to the CDC investigator that Franklin was gripped by an epidemic of "neuromyasthenia." The label aptly covers the syndrome—"neuro" referring to the nervous system, "my" meaning muscles, and "asthenia" indicating weakness. The syndrome observed by Moore and Kirby was a neuromuscular weakness, but the source of the condition was a total mystery.

Neuromyasthenia was first described in 1948 when 450 citizens of Akureyri (Iceland's second-largest city) contracted what originally was thought to be polio. But further examination of the afflicted proved that the polio virus was absent. However, no other viral or bacterial agent could be detected either. By the time of the outbreak in Franklin, twenty similar epidemics, including one at Punta Gorda, Florida, had been reported and still no one had any idea of the cause.

"The general assumption was that a virus was responsible," says Miller. "But nobody really had any hard evidence." Indeed, many speculated that neuromyasthenia attacks were the result of a mass psychosis rather than some physiological illness.

The EIS officer chosen to pursue the cause of the Franklin epidemic was an almost fluke convert to science. "I was a history major as an undergraduate at Harvard," says the slim, bearded Miller, "although my historical interest centered on health. My roommate was a premed and he finally talked me into applying for medical school." During his medical-school years, Miller was asked to write a paper on a subject of scientific research. He duly drafted a report on a newly discovered substance called interferon, currently a hotly pursued possibility for cancer therapy. "Research on that paper led me to an introduction to Dr. James Enders, a well-known virologist. Subsequently I started working with him and became interested in infectious diseases. Once I became fascinated with infectious diseases I realized that the CDC was the perfect place to work on the subject."

Miller recalls, "I arrived in Franklin about two weeks after the peak period of the epidemic, and I immediately visited both the doctors and some of the patients. In most cases the physiological signs of the disease that I saw were much milder than what the local doctors had observed. For example, the first person I examined had become ill ten days before. She initially had trouble with her eye muscles. Several others I saw spoke of being weak in their pelvic regions or leg muscles. But I could not detect any eye-muscle problems in that first patient, nor could I see very obvious signs of weakness in most of the others, although some still showed some mild hand tremors. I was assured that the people I examined had all demonstrated much more severe symptoms.

"To me, at this stage, the physical findings were nowhere near as striking as the psychiatric ones. There was a remarkable inability to concentrate. The people had obvious memory problems. We tried some simple tests, recollecting numbers forward and backward. Some people could do only four numbers forward, three backward—way below what one finds normally.

"At the same time, looking at the medical records, you had to be impressed with the physical problems that had been witnessed before I got to Franklin." One hospital chart describes the experience with a 34-year-old woman, Gloria

Kane (pseudonym), a coil winder for six years. On October 7 while at work, Kane lost some of her sense of balance and she noticed her coordination was poor. She thought the reason might be that she had been standing up for a lengthy period. She sat down at her workbench and was able to finish out the shift. She felt better the next day and even better after a weekend at home. But on Monday after she was on the job for several hours, Kane experienced the same dizziness. She felt "silly" and "walked as though she were drunk."

Kane decided to take the afternoon off, and by evening she had again recovered. Another stint at Potter & Brumfield on Tuesday brought back the disagreeable symptoms. Furthermore, she learned that several co-workers, suffering from similar difficulties, had checked into the hospital. Kane quit work shortly before noon and went to visit her colleagues in the hospital. While there, Gloria Kane's arms and legs suddenly went numb. She fainted. After a blackout of several minutes, she awakened with a severe headache and sharp, stinging pains in her legs. She too was bedded down in the hospital.

Two days later, with her symptoms abated, although the doctors had been unable to diagnose the cause of her sickness, Gloria Kane went home. Shortly afterward, she lapsed into an uncontrollable crying jag, and the numbness returned. Unable to walk, Gloria Kane was readmitted to the hospital.

The medical report on Gloria Kane vividly records her weakness. "She appears ill and somewhat clouded mentally. She gets out of bed by rolling, pushing, and sliding to get to the side of the bed. She rolls her entire body until the right leg touches the floor. Then she pushes her body upright with her hands that are on the bed. All of this is done very slowly."

It was peculiar indeed for a formerly healthy 34-year-old to have suddenly become so feeble she was unable to walk unassisted. However, simply resting in the hospital again seemed to benefit her considerably. Her mind cleared and she slowly regained the power to walk without helping hands or something to lean upon. Yet, more than three weeks after the initial head and neck pains, Gloria Kane still would abruptly break down and cry, and a general malaise prevented her from returning to the job at Potter & Brumfield.

Miller was baffled by cases like that of Gloria Kane. Dr.

William McCormack, another EIS officer, arrived from the CDC in Atlanta to assist in the hunt for an explanation. McCormack had been a student at Downstate Medical School in Brooklyn, New York, and like so many other CDC recruits, faced a military obligation. An obliging professor arranged for him to apply to the CDC. He had signed up with the CDC expecting to spend his two years working on cholera in what was then East Pakistan. "Normally we would have left in August of 1965, but my wife was expecting a child," recalls McCormack, "so we postponed our departure until after the birth. Over Labor Day weekend, however, the war between India and Bangladesh broke out. There was no way I could be sent to the cholera mission. So I hung around Atlanta with nothing to do. To my mind the most awful thing that can happen is to be without anything to pursue, to be bored to death. I begged to be sent out at the first opportunity, and that turned out to be the neuromyasthenia epidemic in Kentucky."

The two CDC agents and the state health department sought to discover the full dimensions of the epidemic. Through newspapers and TV and radio broadcasts and by contacting local doctors and hospitals, they invited anyone with the appropriate symptoms to come to the offices of the state health department for an examination.

"We were concerned that there might be some kind of mass hysteria at work," says McCormack. "Many of the symptoms were the kind you would expect with mass hysteria. There were no laboratory or clinical tests to detect any physiological or organic causes."

The neurological examinations conducted by the two doctors were not terribly helpful. "We had them stand with their eyes closed, arms outstretched, and try to touch their index fingers," says Miller. "They operated well within the normal range. They also did well in the Romberg test, an exercise in which a person touches the heel of one foot to the knee of the other leg and then slides the heel down to the shin. Of course, we were seeing people ten to fourteen days after the beginning of their illness and after their symptoms had begun to disappear. The results suggested no permanent damage, but at the same time we still had no reasons for what actually occurred."

"However," says McCormack, "the circumstances under which we saw the people at the state health department gave us a significant insight. The offices were up a flight of stairs, and layout was such that after we interviewed patients we could, without them knowing it, watch the person go down the steps. Some of them had tremendous difficulty in navigating the stairs. It was obvious that some still had very real muscular weakness."

From all of their sources, Miller and McCormack totaled up fifty-nine people who fitted their case definition of a bona fide victim of the neuromyasthenia epidemic. Of these, forty-nine were employed by Potter & Brumfield, and only one of these was a man. "One of the things that struck me," says Miller, "was that they were almost all women. I kept thinking about any possible reason for females to be so heavily involved."

The routine searches for answers based upon sex were all negative, however. The women had nothing in common in terms of their choices of birth-control medicines, eating habits, or social activities. Food and water were not implicated. The state hygienists had gone over the factory very carefully and could find no signs of infectious agents. None of the processes or materials used at Potter & Brumfield struck them as hazardous. The known chemical toxins that might show up in an industrial atmosphere—trichlorethylene, phosgene, sulfur dioxide, hydrogen sulfide, and carbon monoxide—were not present in amounts sufficient to cause sickness.

"Bill [McCormack] and I constantly talked about the case," recalls Miller. "We figured it was some kind of intoxication but we had no idea what the cause might be. At the time not much attention was being paid to the problems of occupational disease. Everyone was familiar with the chimney sweep's disease [black lung], hatter's disease [mercury poisoning], and a few other classic studies. But there was really very little research, and at the time the CDC itself did not even have a laboratory for the study of toxic substances, or so-called heavy-metal intoxication.

"I decide to call my teacher of occupational medicine at Harvard, Dr. Harriet Hardy, who was also a professor on that subject at Massachusetts Institute of Technology. I told her about the symptoms and she said that among other things it sounded like organic mercury because its effects occurred so fast. Organic mercury is a fat-loving compound. The brain has a lot of fat in it."

This aspect of the hunt for heavy-metal poisoning by the CDC was hampered because the organization had no toxicology lab of its own. Samples had to be sent to another government agency, the Occupational Health and Research Training Facility in Cincinnati.

"We tested the urine specimens for the patients," recalls Miller, "and found higher than normal concentrations of mercury. I sent samples to Harriet Hardy and the results were confirmed. That seemed to indicate the investigation was on the right track. We knew that a majority of the cases came from those working in the coil-winding department of Potter & Brumfield. The rest were either in the assembly or adjusting sections. None of the jobs required the people to handle mercury. So the question was, where did the mercury come from? Dr. Hardy suggested that I consult with a fellow named Richard Chamberlin, an industrial hygienist at MIT."

Chamberlin's expertise in such matters as air-flow currents proved crucial. He suggested that mercury, which was sometimes added to paint, might have vaporized at the Potter & Brumfield factory. Working with Harriet Hardy in some other investigations, Chamberlin previously had discovered the ability of minute amounts of the heavy metal to turn into a gas upon being exposed to heat.

The two EIS officers checked with William Eldred. From him they learned that the electronics plant had been painted in the early summer. Seven different paints were used. The specifications for the paints revealed that two of them contained mercury, added in small amounts by the manufacturers as fungicides. Furthermore, the mercury-infused paint had been extensively used in the coil-winding department, which employed only women, and to some extent in the assembly and adjustment rooms.

Miller and McCormack now sought help from George Boylen, a chemist at MIT. Boylen had developed methods for determining levels for mercury in urine. Now he invented a technique to test the hypothesis that paint actually had vaporized. All of the finishes on the factory furnishings, including the two paints that bore mercury, were applied to a series of wooden panels. After these dried, Chamberlin and Boylen placed them in a sealed glass cylinder. A special instrument measured the mercury vaporization. Even at room temperature, the heavy metal was steadily absorbed into the air. When heat was applied, significantly larger mercury vaporization occurred.

Seven weeks after the initial outbreak in Franklin, Chamberlin calculated the air exchanges in various areas of the factory, then set up devices to capture appropriate samples of the atmosphere. Although the concentrations by this time were relatively low and not significantly toxic, they still exceeded those found in the ordinary air of Cambridge (the home of MIT) by ten times. During the same period, the CDC surveyed mercury levels in urine samples from both people who worked at Potter & Brumfield and Franklin citizens unconnected with the factory or the disease. The levels of mercury of employees in the coil-winding department were significantly higher than those of the remainder of the factory. Incidentally, several people from the assembly unit became sick only after they had temporarily been assigned to coil winding. At least equally telling, paint from another production area contained no mercury. Not a single person from there developed neuromyasthenia.

Miller and McCormack now wrestled with questions of why the mercury poisoning suddenly erupted in the early autumn and with such fury in the coil-winding department. The answers were disarmingly simple and lay in the seasonal changes of climate. Checking records for operations in the factory, the investigators learned that in the assembly rooms where some of the earlier cases had broken out, management turned on space heaters to cut the chill of cool days that came in late September. That heat was sufficient to act upon the mercury in the paint. In the coil-winding department, the deadly paint had been applied not only to the walls but also to the steam conduits that led from a boiler to the heating units in the department. The steam conduits were subject to much more intensive heat, the extra temperature throwing off higher increments of mercury into the air breathed by the employees. The greatest number of cases dated from the very first day that Potter & Brumfield began pumping steam through the conduits of its coil-winding department.

There seemed little doubt that the mystery of Franklin's neuromyasthenia epidemic was solved, except there were those ten cases of people who had never entered the works at Potter & Brumfield and, therefore could not have been exposed to the gasified mercury.

"It's true," says McCormack, "that it wasn't conclusively proven. But what was important was that the rates were so much higher at the factory, forty-nine cases among the 700 people who worked for Potter & Brumfield, compared to only ten people in the rest of the 11,000 living in the community. Also, we were dealing with a clinical definition of an illness, which is at best imprecise. It's not as if we had a bacteriological culture we could identify in a lab."

Miller, seventeen years after his sojourn in Franklin, says, "There's a very outside chance that it was all a red herring, the mercury vaporization. However, a lot of things that are classified as psychological symptoms are related to organic or toxic events. Even with flu there is a postinfection asthenia [weakness] when the person feels unable to get up, to work. More and more psychiatrists are focusing on organic causes for mental problems. Sure it might have been mass hysteria." Miller pauses. "Except there was that mercury in the paint, there were higher levels in the victims, and the experiments by Chamberlin and Boylen showed how it could happen."

But still, what about those ten cases of people who were never in Potter & Brumfield? As McCormack suggested, diagnosis of neuromyasthenia is less than exact or conclusive. Three of these victims, however, had previous histories of what they said was diagnosed as a "nervous breakdown." Another had a sister hospitalized with psychosis. All but one of the remainder had close contact with people working at Potter & Brumfield. Mass hysteria, while seemingly an unlikely candidate for explaining the entire epidemic, might well be the source of these ten cases.

Altogether, Miller was to make four extended visits to Franklin, and in the course of his hunt he might have been discouraged had it not been for the encouragement of Alexander Langmuir, then in his final year as chief of epidemiology at the CDC. "He was a powerful, intellectual personality, an indefatigable worker," says Miller, "and he kept in touch with everything going on." Miller still retains copies of his reports on the epidemic with Langmuir's handwritten comments appended.

"Langmuir made us feel that the work of the epidemiologist was paramount. There had to be specimens collected by someone in the field if a lab was to pin down the cause. There is no way a university can do this kind of work, nor any private organization. It isn't basic research but very practical work. But there also had to be a lab able to find the responsible agent."

Looking back on the triumph, George Miller says, "I think Harriet Hardy was the real hero. She's the one who fingered the cause."

But at the time, Miller, McCormack, and Chamberlin received the recognition. The paper the EIS doctors submitted to the CDC some months later won the Langmuir prize. (The founder of the EIS having retired to teach at Harvard, the CDC had established an award for the best research by EIS officers.) David Sencer, who succeeded Langmuir, recognized the importance of the work on neuromyasthenia for the CDC. Says Miller, "He told me then, 'This investigation opens a new chapter in the kinds of investigations for the CDC.'" Subsequently the Occupational Health and Research Training Facility in Cincinnati became the National Institute for Occupational Safety and Health (NIOSH), and an integral part of the CDC. Toxicologists and a lab equipped to screen for and probe the effects of toxins began a massive effort to track health problems generated by poisonous substances and pollution.

Bill McCormack shipped out to Bangladesh for a two-and-a-half-year tour with an anti-cholera team. Upon his return, he served at several medical installations before taking a post back at Downstate, where he now concerns himself with sexually transmitted maladies, including several cases of the gay men's disease (see Chapter 4). "Those cases involve an enormous amount of time and effort," he remarks. He leans to the theory that sexual promiscuity is the key.

"The EIS was a fabulous experience," says George Miller. "It's like being an intern, when every patient you see is sick or dying. It's only when you start to practice medicine that you see well people. It was so exciting. I thought nothing of getting on a plane to some far-off place every week. I was in Africa when my son was being born, somewhere else when our second child came. I frequently left my wife home with the two small kids. When you're young, in your 20s, you do that. It was, after all, a very heady thing to fly to Africa and the very first thing on arrival, meet with the U.S. ambassador to the country.

"As a training system, I think the EIS is unequaled. The people of my EIS class have made incredible contributions." But eventually the intoxicating adventures of a disease detective had to come to an end. And as if aware that no job in medicine could compete with that exhilarating experience, Miller dramatically changed his orientation. "I ended up with more interest in the lab than in field work." Toward that end he is now Enders Professor in Pediatric Infectious Diseases at Yale University Medical School. (The chair is in honor of the man who influenced Miller to devote himself to the study of infection.)

All of the Franklin victims of neuromyasthenia recovered completely. The CDC's discoveries in Kentucky were among the first to find explanations for those epidemics of neuromuscular weakness that had sudden puzzled medicine, beginning with the outbreak in Iceland. In fact, the disease of neuromyasthenia is no longer a vague mystery associated with an unknown virus or mass psychosis. After a brief life in the literature of medicine, neuromyasthenia itself disappeared.

CHAPTER
——13——

The Circling Disease

In May 1981, Dr. Robert Bortolussi, a specialist in pediatric infections at Dalhousie University Medical School, Halifax, Nova Scotia, was asked to look in on a premature baby. The infant was in pitiable condition, gasping for breath in an isolette, with a severe infection. The exact nature of the preemie's distress could not be immediately determined through Bortolussi's clinical observations. "It could have been a Group B strep infection," says Bortolussi, "or a number of other things. The only way to find out was through laboratory examination of blood and tissue specimens."

While life-support apparatus labored, futilely as it turned out, to keep the neonate breathing, technicians drew their samples and prepared cultures. Some twenty-four hours later, Bortolussi received the disquieting news. The child had suffered from listeriosis. "Ordinarily," says Bortolussi, "I would see at most two cases of listeriosis in a year. This was the fourth for the month of May alone."

Listeriosis, named for the great British scientist Joseph Lister, who pioneered the notion of antiseptic surgery, is a product of *Listeria monocytogenes*, a bacterium that lives in soil, water, and vegetation. It is classified as a zoonosis, because it is relatively common among animals and birds. Since some afflicted animals tend to move around and around, listeriosis is popularly known as the circling disease.

While the sickness has been considered mainly a problem for veterinarians, it occasionally is transmitted to humans. Just as it does with cattle and sheep, listeriosis may affect the human brain and the membranes that surround the heart and stomach. It is particularly threatening to newborns whose mothers contract the disease shortly before giving birth. Listeriosis is the third most common cause of bacterial meningitis and takes a deadly toll in spontaneous abortions, stillbirths, and birth defects. In the infant who was the fourth victim in May 1981, *Listeria monocytogenes* had produced a particularly devastating septic illness termed granulomatosis infantiscepticum.

"We had investigators from the Canadian Laboratory Centre for Disease Control in Ottawa looking into the matter for two weeks," says Bortolussi, "but they were mystified. They had distributed questionnaires to the people involved, but nothing offered any indications of where the disease was coming from. Over the years, I had had informal contact with the CDC in Atlanta on a number of matters. I thought maybe they could do some of the lab work for us and at the same time give us some advice on conducting an epidemiological study."

Among those attached to the Special Pathogens Branch of the CDC at the time Bortolussi telephoned Atlanta was Dr. Walter Schlech III. An EIS officer, he had already achieved some distinction by dint of his phone survey which compiled the data that pinpointed the RELY tampon as a prominent factor in the outbreak of toxic shock syndrome (see Chapter 6). Slim, medium in height, and mustachioed, Schlech remembers the discussion with Bortolussi. "Bob was very concerned; listeriosis was occurring in 1 percent of the live births at the hospital and actually by the end of May he had seen ten documented cases in roughly thirty days. He asked if we would do some of the serotyping on specimens. We said we'd be happy to help out but that we'd also like the opportunity to make an epidemiological investigation."

The bargain was easily struck, and Schlech soon arrived in Halifax. His initial effort was to ascertain the true extent of the problem, whether it was only in the Halifax area, or infecting the Maritime Provinces that include Nova Scotia, or even spreading across all of Canada. Letters were dispatched to physicians notifying them of the outbreak of listeriosis and soliciting information from them about possible cases. The result was the discovery of several more victims in the provinces of Prince Edward Island and New Brunswick. Information of this nature confirmed that listeriosis was cropping up throughout the Maritime area. While not confined to Halifax it was also not a nationwide threat.

Says Schlech, "We also reviewed the records for admissions on stillbirths and spontaneous abortions at Grace Maternity Hospital, the only place of that kind in Halifax, and at Victoria General, which provides more than half of the acute-care beds in the city. We asked the Nova Scotia Provincial Laboratory for its records on any evidence of increased incidence of mononucleosis, since some earlier research suggested that *Listeria monocytogenes* may produce a syndrome very much akin to that of infectious mononucleosis."

The epidemiological survey organized by Schlech covered the period 1979 to 1981. It indicated thirty-four cases of perinatal listeriosis and seven infections in adults clustered between the beginning of March and the start of September 1981. The peak period was during the summer months, but a graph of the epidemic plotted the increase in incidence during the previous year. While there was apparently no detectable shift in the spontaneous-abortion rate in Halifax, the toll was high. Five women lost their babies before birth, four more were stillborn. In twenty-three cases a seriously ill child, usually premature, was diagnosed as a listeriosis victim. Only two kids were perfectly healthy at birth even though their mothers were subsequently found to have had listeriosis. More than 25 percent of the infants born with the infection died, in spite of the most aggressive supportive care and antibiotics.

The disease was rough on adults too. While many of the pregnant women exhibited the kinds of symptoms associated with a flu attack shortly before the birth of their children, there were seven instances of listeriosis in six men and one woman who was not pregnant. Two of these individuals also succumbed to the disease.

Schlech, with the assistance of public health nurses in Nova Scotia, collected a wealth of information on the victims as well as more laboratory specimens. "All the victims were asked about their medical history," says Schlech, "where they lived, the kind of work they did, the travel they experienced. We kept looking for the common thread, something to explain how the particular individual came to be exposed to listeria. We also gathered a general food history and then looked at particular items—the brand names, the special foods that might provide a clue. It's always been assumed that listeriosis can be transmitted from an animal reservoir to humans, but with two exceptions, no one ever demonstrated the actual pathways. Veterinarians delivering infected calves have come down with the illness, and one study in England reported that a baby had contracted the disease after drinking milk from a sick cow."

What had been expected to be a short visit to Nova Scotia for Schlech had become a long-term assignment as the mystery of the source continued. He did not find his stay onerous, however. "As a kid I had done a lot of moving around. My father was in the service, a rear admiral eventually in submarines. Nova Scotia was among the nicer places I had seen." As a matter of fact, Schlech had seen some of the world at its worst. He graduated from high school during the mid-1960s. As the son of a military man he did not think in the same terms as some of those who eventually became his colleagues at the CDC. Schlech actually volunteered during the Vietnam War. He chose, naturally, the navy.

"I figured I would be a hospital corpsman, get a cushy job in some Stateside hospital, and then go to medical school. I hadn't realized that since the marines do not have their own corpsmen, the navy supplies them. I found myself in Vietnam, attached to the marines in combat. I was there for 1967–68; it was a harrowing experience, going through the Tet offensive and being at Kasan during the long siege."

Fortunately, he emerged from Vietnam unscathed. After med school he signed up for an infectious-disease fellowship in Nashville. "Bill Shaffner, a very outgoing academic physician who'd been in the EIS, told me I'd be a natural for the CDC," recalls Schlech. "Actually I had no experience with epidemiology in medical school, but I applied and was accepted." Thus the old-boy network recruited another candidate.

In Nova Scotia, Schlech routinely continued to check out foods that might bear the bacteria. Then he received an unexpected break. One of the latest listeriosis patients was an 81-year-old man who had just arrived in Halifax on a visit.

"He was of great interest to me because he had immigrated to Halifax, coming from a place where there was no history of listeriosis infections. His experience might reveal something we had overlooked."

Schlech patiently quizzed the elderly man, who was slowly recovering from pneumonia as a result of his bout with listeriosis. "I asked him particularly about what he had eaten in Halifax. He told me that the remains were still all in the refrigerator of the apartment he was using. I gave him six bucks for everything in it and had it all examined in the lab. There was one new item: cole slaw. While the technicians attempted to culture something from the cole slaw, we went back to the other victims and asked them if they had eaten that same food. The answer was yes in many instances."

When the examination of the slaw retrieved from the refrigerator uncovered *Listeria monocytogenes* among the cabbage leaves, Schlech now endeavored to trace the source of the bacteria. "I went to the manufacturing plant and talked to the people who ran it. It was obvious that there was no contamination in the processing; the bacteria had to have come from the raw materials. The problem was that there were many different farmers who sold cabbage to the processor."

Interviewing all of the growers and testing their crops would be a long-drawn-out affair. Then Schlech came up with a shortcut. He obtained a list of those farmers whom veterinarians in the Maritime Provinces had listed as having listeriosis in their livestock. Among the names, Schlech discovered one farmer who also supplied the cabbage to the cole slaw dealer.

"I went to his farm," says Schlech, "and after visiting with him awhile learned he was a bit different in the way he did things. He used raw manure from his sheep to fertilize the fields. Most farmers steam their manure first and then spread it, because the steam destroys weed seeds. As a side effect, the treatment would also have killed bacteria such as listeria. But this fellow did not believe in treating the manure. Furthermore, after the October harvest, he stored the cabbage in a shed over the winter, into the early spring. Listeria happens to be one of those rare organisms that actually prefers low temperatures." Thus, over the dark, frigid months before the crop went to market, with the thermometer hovering just above freezing, the colonies of *Listeria monocytogenes* propagated among the stored cabbages. Nothing in the processing of the food subsequently would have interfered with the growth of the bacteria and its ability to infect. The origins of the epidemic and its pathway were clear.

Schlech had worked all along with Bortolussi and other health professionals in Halifax. "We were all very impressed with his demeanor," says Bortolussi, "and the way he went about things. We had been looking for a person to serve as an epidemiologist, and after Wally finished the investigation we offered him the post."

With his EIS term running out, Schlech accepted the offer. "I had such a good time up here," he remarked shortly after he took up permanent abode in Halifax. "I've got a wife and two small kids; we bought a home in a place where the kids can run up and down the street without anything to worry about.

"Professionally, there's a lot going on, and the territory is wide open for an epidemiologist. They haven't done much investigating previously and just haven't had the resources to tease out things and to follow up. The work at the CDC was fun; I enjoyed it and met some interesting people. Now I'm in virgin territory and the work combines clinical duties along with the opportunities for investigations."

Thus the circling disease led one man to a home.

CHAPTER
14

Investigations for
the Future

READING THE *Morbidity and Mortality Weekly Report (MMWR)*, scanning the EIS officers' accounts of their investigations (called EPI 2s), skimming the entire report production of the CDC, one draws an uneasy sense of a universe teeming with malevolence, microscopic organisms hell-bent on the destruction of humans. The truth is quite the contrary. In spite of the fact that a square inch of human skin hosts a thick zoo of microbes, intersection of people with health-threatening bugs is an accident and often is as damaging to the organisms as to their much larger victims.

The sheer numbers for infectious-disease cases indicate the vast job still ahead. For example, chicken pox strikes more than 100,000 a year. Tuberculosis still infects about 30,000 annually. Flu figures vary widely from year to year, but they can soar into the millions. The venereal threats have been on a rampage—80,000 cases of syphilis, 500,000 of gonorrhea, 500,000 of genital herpes—all new victims each year. The 200,000 cases of hepatitis B include 200 deaths from acute infection; another 280 persons succumb to liver cancer directly resulting from hepatitis, and 3,500 die from cirrhosis caused by the type B virus.

Legionnaires' disease filled the newspapers in 1976, but only a year before, there were an estimated 544,000 infections of St. Louis encephalitis in the United States. Each year, about 18,000 people come down with bacterial meningitis, with perhaps 2,500 deaths as a consequence. When someone toted up the cost of the yearly infections of this bacterial meningitis, it came to $58 million. Indeed, the infectious diseases wreak a staggering $6 billion worth of hospital costs for the approximately 27 million patient days of acute hospital care each year.

These are some of the more common infections, but the CDC is kept busy with small but very intense fires of infection.

Consider, for example, the rickettsiae, those creatures that fall somewhere between bacteria and viruses. Something over 1,200 incidences of rickettsial disease, mostly Rocky Mountain spotted fever, are reported to the CDC annually (undoubtedly quite a few more cases occur but go either unreported or undiagnosed). That may not seem like much of a threat to 220 million Americans, but to the 1,200 victims (thirty deaths) the rickettsiae are hardly a minor matter. Joe McDade of legionella fame (see Chapter 2) need not fear a slump in his field of expertise.

Even rarer is something known as primary amoebic meningoencephalitis (PAM)—swimmer's disease. It strikes people bathing in freshwater lakes or ponds, and there have been less than a dozen cases recorded in the past few years. However, it is almost inevitably fatal. Public announcement of a single case is enough to set the phones ringing at the CDC as anxious citizens worry about the risk to those headed for the local swimming hole. So far, the CDC has been unable either to detect the source or to determine treatment for the deadly neurological symptoms that begin within a few days after infection. But the matter of PAM remains a CDC project if only in terms of tissue specimens on file in its storehouse of slides.

Several thousand rabies cases come to the attention of the CDC every year. Fortunately, only a handful of humans are infected; experts in zoonoses find rabies in skunks, bats, raccoons, foxes, flying squirrels, and such exotic animals as mongooses and minks. As humans invade the habitats of even the most feral animals, the risks of rabies increase. A few years ago, an Alaska pipeline worker spotted a distressed caribou. The animal was behaving bizarrely; it had collapsed after an abortive run at a highway sign. When the samaritan attempted to soothe the beast, his hands became covered with blood and saliva from its mouth and nostrils. Then the caribou turned on him, and he narrowly escaped its charge. Subsequent examination revealed the presence of rabies in the animal; the would-be savior required antirabial treatment.

An even stranger, more terrifying case involved a 37-year-old Boise, Idaho, woman who died of rabies. Seven weeks before her death she had received a corneal transplant donated by a man from Baker, Oregon. He had succumbed to what was diagnosed as Guillain-Barre syndrome, a rare neurological infection (its incidence increased sharply during the swine flu immunization program and brought that effort to an end) that weakens, even paralyzes, victims.

After her transplant the woman made satisfactory progress for about a month until she developed a headache over her right eye. The pain worsened and then paralysis slowly spread from her face to the rest of her body. She died in eight days. An autopsy revealed rabies. The source had to be the donor, although an intensive investigation could not find any animal bites on his body. However, like plague victim John Bigbee (see Chapter 11), he was a lumber worker, which conceivably exposed him to animal-borne agents. Furthermore, his avocation was trapping, shooting, and skinning coyotes, which made him at some risk of contact with infected wildlife.

Often, as in this rabies case, the CDC disease detectives can do little more than discover how something happened. The victim is beyond help; the killer has made its escape undetected. At best, publication of the facts of an investigation can perhaps induce precautions for warding off future infections. Presumably, the tale of the rabies-infected cornea will mean more searching studies on the cause of death in prospective organ donors.

Then there are those ongoing mysteries, ones that run up against a blank, unyielding wall leaving the identity of the killer unknown. Such has been the experience of Dr. Roy Baron, whose early experiences with the CDC sent him to Africa in search of the Ebola virus (see Chapter 10).

The investigation began about 3,000 miles from Atlanta. Dr. Steven Helgerson, a psychiatrist who did his undergraduate work at the University of Puget Sound and then went on to earn his medical degree and a master's in public health at the University of Washington, signed on as an epidemic intelligence officer in 1980. Like so many of his colleagues in the CDC, Helgerson had been involved in a number of projects abroad, working in Europe, Japan, Hong Kong, and the

Philippines. To his delight, the EIS had posted him back to the Northwest, as a field service officer working at the Oregon Department of Human Resources.

One night he was invited to have dinner at the home of the state epidemiologist, Dr. John A. Googins. It was a stimulating evening, for among the guests were Dr. Googins's son, also named John, who had been in the Peace Corps and now worked as a counselor in a welfare clinic with Southeast Asians settled in the area.

In the course of the evening, the younger Googins mentioned a persistent rumor among some of the local refugees, the Hmong mountain people from Laos. There was a good deal of anxiety among them because of the talk about strange nighttime deaths of men 25 to 40 years of age in their beds. Helgerson checked out the rumor and learned that it was true; there had been several such mysterious deaths among the Hmong.

Some 1,500 miles away, Dr. Michael Osterholm, the Minnesota state epidemiologist who played an important role in the case of toxic shock syndrome (see Chapter 6), had also heard of mysterious deaths among Hmong refugees. A local physician reported to Osterholm about the death of one of his patients for no apparent reason. Osterholm then began to check around, and suddenly he too discovered that there were four such deaths in his area.

The CDC gradually became more aware of the bizarre health problems among the Hmong. After Dr. Larry Lewman, the coroner from Multnomah County, had done his second autopsy in two days on young, presumably healthy men who died suddenly in their sleep and could not find any explanation for their deaths, he notified local refugee authorities. Dixie Cole, the refugee coordinator for the Health and Human Services group in the region, subsequently notified the CDC, and an investigation began. Dr. Andrew Vernon was appointed to lead the probe. Shortly thereafter, Dr. Roy Baron volunteered for the project.

Says Baron, "We looked at medical examiners' files to see how frequently an ME who does an autopsy on an apparent natural death doesn't come up with an answer for the cause. We found it is very uncommon but in a space of close to four years, we could now find more than twenty such deaths among Hmong between the ages of 25 and 47, and that is five or six times greater than one finds among our indigenous population." (Subsequently, early in 1982, the total of mysterious deaths among the Hmong was pegged at thirty-nine.) The MEs did all of the possible tests including toxicological screens to find any kind of poison, but no unusual findings showed.

Sitting in a sub-basement office of the CDC in Atlanta, the youthful-looking Baron played with his pipe and said, "You feel you're so close, as if you're not asking the right question, and then you wonder maybe we'll never know. If someone would tell you the right answer, then maybe you would kick yourself for not having thought of it."

In the cubicle opposite Baron, his motorcycle helmet the one colorful item on his desk, Andrew Vernon confessed, "This is not going to be an easy nut to crack. We've had some spurts of optimism. When Roy went to Oregon to examine the pathology specimens, there had been some minor abnormalities in heart tissue which alone would not seem a likely cause of death, but at least it offered a common thread. But a pathology review showed that these abnormalities as a cause of death were not borne out."

Roy Baron and others organized a series of painstaking interviews with all of the family members who had had contact with the dead men. At the same time, scientists restudied the tissues of the deceased in search of some significant changes in pathology which might have been overlooked. An effort was made to survey the death certificates of all Indo-Chinese refugees since 1975.

There was some evidence that at least two of the victims had not been deep in sleep at the time of their deaths. In one instance, a woman spoke to her husband and within a few minutes she found him lying lifeless in his bed. In a second case, a couple were awakened by the sound of a crying child. While the wife went to fetch a bottle, she left the baby in her husband's arms. She returned to find the infant lying on the floor, her husband dead on the bed.

A year later, Vernon left for the staff of the Emory Medical School and Baron assumed command of the investigation. "So far," says Baron, "we're on a fishing expedition. We're not sure where to start or to look." The epidemiological study

involves sifting through the compilations of all details of previous illnesses, where the victims were born, when they left
Laos, how much time they spent as refugees, their occupations in Laos, their military experience—anything that might
indicate some kind of event that the victims had in common.
There has been much speculation about stress, and the epidemiological surveys include information on the lives of family members, the circumstances under which members have
died, socioeconomic status past and current, and even the
ability to speak English. For every victim, three "controls"—
southeast Asian refugees—have also been interviewed. Dietary
changes have been studied; an intensive search has been made
for any kind of physical or emotional symptoms in the two
weeks prior to death. To date, in Baron's words, "nothing
has fallen out."

The pathology studies, according to Baron, have been of an
exhaustive nature, and tissue samples of the stilled hearts
were submitted to cardiologists. The most hotly pursued
answer has to do with the conduction system of the heart.
Examination of this tissue is a highly technical, laborious,
specialized procedure. Rarely is medicine called upon to study
a death so minutely. The signs of death ordinarily are far
grosser, more easily identified.

Says Baron, "The question is also, if indeed there has been
some strange malfunction in the conduction system, what
could have triggered it? What had brought on these 'electrical
accidents,' as some have called them? What makes a heart
more excitable? We are aware that nearly every death occurred
during sleep—that seems to be more than a chance occurrence. What happens in the sleep process—another area for
study."

The Hmong themselves add a note of mystery to the case.
They lived in a near Stone Age existence in the mountains of
Laos until the war in Vietnam infected their homeland. Within the space of a few years, this primitive (in Western terms)
people was thrust into twentieth-century technology and id-
eologies. It was perhaps the most violent uprooting of a
people in history.

Lab tests and comparisons with other Laotian refugees
eliminated a number of possible causes of the sleeping death
—such as opium grown and used in Laos but not here, any

known viral agents, diet or nutritional background. Further
investigation revealed that other Asians—notably Filipino
and Japanese men—have died under similar circumstances.
The Filipino syndrome is known as *bangungut*, which means
"nightmare" and was so dubbed because the sounds uttered
just before death resembled those of a person caught up in
a wild dream. But there is no explanation of why a vivid nightmare should kill a handful of Asiatic men.

Who among us has not awakened one night with heart
pounding, body sweating from a cascade of frightening images
more horrible than described in the cool literature of the good
Dr. Freud? Yet death from nightmare or anything similar
has never been reported in the annals of American medicine,
at least until the Hmong settled here. There are no medical
records to tell whether such an event was part of Hmong life
before the war.

The one survivor of the syndrome, 36-year-old Ge Xiong
of Seattle, has been thoroughly examined and his sleep patterns watched for some clues about his breathing, eye movements (rapid eye movements are associated with dreams),
brain waves, and heart rhythm. So far the experts have been
unable to link his sleep physiology with his close encounter
with death.

In 1982, Baron was still on the case and was quoted as
saying, "We've actually got some results that I think are
substantive." But whatever they were he has refused to dis-
close them until all studies were completed, all avenues ex-
hausted. And Baron or a successor will stay on the case until
it is solved—just as the mysteries of St. Elizabeth's Hospital
and Pontiac fever were solved eventually.

The investigation into the nighttime deaths may prove to
be something entirely apart from the early medical detection
efforts of the CDC. But even if it proves to be ethnic, genetic, or emotional, the war of the CDC against communicable diseases will probably never end. Bacteria, viruses, and
rickettsiae are as comfortable on our planet as any other living
cells. They were here before mankind and will probably
endure even after higher forms of life vanish because of some
cosmic incident or self-made bang. Furthermore, old diseases
such as leprosy, develop a resistance to drugs, forcing experts
like Charles Shepherd to continue to battle them. New

scourges like dengue fever, now marching from the tropic climes to the Caribbean Islands and making menacing ges- tuers toward the continental U.S., appear with depressing regularity.

But the CDC's charter now includes diseases that might not be considered communicable in the traditional meaning of a human who accidentally passes his or her germs to an- other. Instead, illnesses frequently have been stimulated, un- wittingly, by humans or even created by medical experts— physical or emotional disorders that are iatrogenic or due to the treatment. Even in the great health centers where gigantic efforts to heal are made, diseases are often fostered.

A hospital is a place people go for the diagnosis and cure of a disease. And as a country rich in its tradition of high- quality care for the acutely ill (and somewhat less renowned for its attention to preventive care), the U.S. has 7,000 acute- care hospitals with more than one million beds. These are occupied by 37,200,000 bodies annually, and on any given day one can count 800,000 people in the country spending time as a hospitalized patient.

But hospitals can be very dangerous for sick people. About 5 percent of those who enter a hospital will become infected with some disease they did not have at the time of admission. That adds up to 40,000 cases of new illnesses, among the daily population in the institutions where people go to be cured. Such diseases are called nosocomial infections.

Hospitals have a high risk of infecting patients for several reasons. Many of the patients have infectious conditions which may spread to others. Second, because the diseases that resulted in admission reduce normal resistance, the hospital popula- tion is often extremely vulnerable to second infections. Fur- thermore, the nature of the institutions, where the staff works in close proximity to sick people and moves among them, and where so many people are packed into a confined area, pro- vides a favorable environment for the outbreak of disease.

Dr. Jim Allen, chief of the CDC's Hospital Infections Branch, rattles off the statistics with the air of a man who accepts the problem as inevitable. "You can't eliminate risk from a hospital, but you can hope to control the amount of infections. It's our job to assist hospitals in dealing with unusual problems as well as discovering procedures that reduce risk."

Dr. Allen's association with public health has a touch of genetics. "My father was a doctor who worked for a precursor to the Agency for International Development in India. He also did research on the medical effects of the atomic-bomb explosions. I started out as a pediatrician. When the choice came down to going to Vietnam or serving as an EIS officer, I opted for Atlanta."

As an example of hospital infections, Allen cites a nosocomial disease that ravaged a large hospital in a Southern city. "They reported a cluster of patients in intensive care who developed a blood-borne infection," says Dr. Allen. "There were a number of deaths. The pathology reports immediately indicated an infection by a bacterium called *Serratia marcescens*. Most of the problems we run into in hospitals are bacterial; occasionally one will come across a viral or fungal outbreak. It is almost never a parasitic attack"—which is a testament to at least rudimentary sanitary procedures.

Serratia marcescens is a small, ubiquitous, rod-shaped organism characterized by a red pigment that shows up when the bacterium is cultured in a laboratory at room temperature. As a member of bacteria's bacilli family, *Serratia marcescens* has the ability to form spores within its cells. These retain all of the genetic material of the microbe and serve as a dormant form of the bacillus. The spores tend to be resistant to heat, cold, and drying, which makes an organism like *Serratia marcescens* difficult to eliminate without obliterating many other living organisms in a human body. Nor would one want to engage in a blanket destruction of all bacteria. The human body employs a great many bacteria for its own use. Dr. Allen points out that the normal bacteria in the bowels prevent diarrhea. Bacteria present on the skin check the pervasive alpha streptococci, the source of sore throats.

"Even though infections at hospitals, like this one [at the Southern hospital] involving the surgery patients, come from very familiar bacteria," explains Dr. Allen, "more and more frequently it proves to be a bacterium that is resistant to even multiple antibiotic attack." Control of such an infection lies not so much in finding the proper drugs to treat the patients as in locating the means by which they are becoming infected.

In search of the source of the *Serratia marcescens*, Dr. Allen and others probed into every crevice, orifice, and corner of the patients' and staffs' bodies that might harbor the bacteria. "I swabbed skins, ears, groins, cultured stools and sputum, even took scrapings under toenails," recalls Dr. Allen.

"Once we began to investigate the matter and studied the hospital records, we also realized that this was far more widespread than the hospital staff realized. The infections had been going on longer than anyone there was aware of. Furthermore, it had also appeared in another part of the hospital." The culprit was known but the critical question remained: Who was the accomplice—human, animal or mechanical—which enabled *Serratia marcescens* to go about its deadly business?

The CDC investigator studied the routines in the hospital. No single, obvious source of infection was discovered. The solution was to insist upon more rigorous conformity to simple sanitary requirements—hand washing, using sterilized gowns and gloves when dressing wounds. The epidemic was halted. "If people did what they should do all of the time," remarks Allen, "we'd reduce 20 percent of the background of infections, and that would be more significant than dealing with the peaks and clusters of infection in a hospital. Infection is a part of life. Pull a hundred people off the street at random, you will find twenty of them harboring staph aureus bacteria [the germ behind toxic shock syndrome] in their noses, throats, or vaginas."

In another large hospital, a high percentage of patients who had received cardiac surgery developed blood-borne infections. Several died, and this serratia infection was a contributing factor to the deaths. The investigators learned that unlike the general run of patients at the hospital, all of these individuals were constantly checked for blood pressure by means of a tube directly inserted into one of their arteries and hooked up to a blood-pressure-monitoring machine. The hospital had sought to save money by cleaning and resterilizing the equipment. Unfortunately, there were inevitable breaks in the device's membranes. Bacteria took up residence there and survived in spite of the routine sterilization procedures.

Once the hospital authorities were persuaded to follow the protocol and dispose of disposable items, the epidemic ended. Similarly, the CDC looked into a peritoneal dialysis unit that was constantly troubled by infections of the peritoneum (an area of the stomach through which an artificial blood-cleansing system can be operated). Again the machines proved to be the source of the contamination. The disinfection techniques between patients were inadequate.

Nosocomial infections are unlikely to disappear as a major problem. Allen points out, "People are prone to error, new procedures are constantly developed, the equipment changes rapidly, there is tremendous turnover in personnel. Making sure they know all the ins and outs is an enormous job. The maintenance people are often critical to the prevention of infection, yet their general level of education and training is not very good. We're lucky we don't have bigger problems. Night shifts are often understaffed. The more complicated procedures and machines, the more than can go wrong." Hospitals are also reluctant to call in the CDC, to let out the word that they have a nosocomial epidemic, because that encourages the appearance of what Allen calls "the sharks," litigators in search of lawsuits for negligence.

Hospitals remain one of the growth industries in the United States even as the economy appears to flag. Americans have come to expect the acute-care institutions to provide ever more sophisticated therapy—which, as Allen notes, bears with it higher risks of secondary infections. In addition, with the population aging and more and more people surviving the traditional old killer diseases, a much larger number of individuals require extended or even permanent residency in a therapeutic environment. These citizens are quite vulnerable to nosocomial problems. The CDC can expect to be increasingly involved with this type of problem.

The CDC's investment in prevention services has long been an intensive one. This section of the CDC gobbles up a substantial percentage of the agency's funds and employs many professions.

For example, Dr. Timothy Nolan, a pediatrician and former EIS officer, was in charge of the CDC's anti-flu program for several years. "There are three basic types of flu—A, B, C," says Nolan. "The first two, A and B, are of epidemic potential and of concern to public health. Under A and B there are many subtypes, and generally they each require a different kind of immunization. The types change because of bio-chemical differences that will make the genetic material in an A differ from a B or C. They all behave differently. Type C is rarely involved in a major outbreak of illness. A large por-tion of the population has antibodies to the Type C strain, and when the disease shows, it's mild and even subclinical [unnoticeable in children].

"The B pattern is marked by sporadic outbreaks through the year. It tends to be more prevalent among school-age kids, although in '79–'80 we had an epidemic that struck all age groups with higher mortality than usual.

"It's the A forms that are the ones we usually talk about— Hong Kong, Asian, and swine, for example. We actually didn't misidentify swine flu during that period of '75–'76 [just before Legionnaires' disease appeared]. The strains we iso-lated in New Jersey were swine flu, all right, but the question that couldn't be answered was whether they were identical to that of the 1918 version which killed 500,000 people in the U.S., 20 million around the world. It was only in the late 1930s that we learned how to grow viruses. We just didn't have anything from 1918 to match and positively identify the specimens from 1975–76. The antibodies we had from peo-ple who had survived the epidemic in 1918 did react. We had to go on that evidence. But you can have similar antibodies and still have a different disease."

The CDC's flu immunization program tries to determine in advance the subtype of flu most likely to appear in a com-ing year. "We do it by looking at the cases which have been most prevalent toward the end of the previous year," says the tall, slender Nolan. "But there's not tremendous accuracy in such predictions. Sometimes changes occur at the end of the season and we may miss them. In evaluating the coming threats, the CDC relies on information from those coping with epidemics, upon research in state institutions, its own labs, and the World Health Organization. All of these focus on a flu specimen looking for clues to what's likely to be domi-nant."

As a case in point, the first flu in the 1978–79 season broke out in a junior high school near Los Angeles. The information from physicians and labs doing throat swabs indicated that the isolates were close to the Brazilian flu, an A type. Based on this data, the CDC pushed for the production of A-Brazil-type vaccine. It was a good guess. The right vaccine was manufactured and distributed, the flu's attack limited.

The struggles against the flu are unlikely to abate. The varieties in flu viruses are so numerous that it will be necessary to maintain at least the current level of vigilance merely in order to keep the disease at bay, to say nothing of conquering it.

However, in another arena, the CDC is almost ready to declare itself the winner. Measles—rubella, as it's known in the health trade—has almost been eradicated as a domestic disease.

In most states, measles cases must be reported by any physician treating an infection. But there has always been some doubt about the reporting efficiency. Many doctors don't want to bother with additional paperwork, particularly when it concerns what appears to be a minor problem. Dr. Walter Orenstein, the current chief of the Immunization Division (and the first EIS man posted to Philadelphia during the Legionnaires' disease epidemic), points out that the last measles pandemic of 1964–65 listed 450,000 cases. "It may be that the actual incidence was closer to 4.5 million," suggests Dr. Orenstein. The most recent epidemic in the U.S. in 1977 had 57,345 cases reported. For 1981, the total number of cases was less than 5,000. For 1982, the figures are about half that. "Our aim, at present," says the bearded Orenstein, "is the eradication and elimination of perpetual transmission in the United States. I suppose," he adds, "my specialty of pediatrics has made me more oriented to preventive medicine."

Measles is only occasionally life-threatening. However, a measles infection frequently leaves the body so weakened that more dangerous enemies such as encephalitis and meningitis may invade with relative impunity. In any event, the cost of a measles epidemic is sizable. Nurse epidemiologist Barbara Olson surveyed an outbreak at a high school in Arizona and found that the forty-four cases added up to a total loss of $12,166. The sum covers doctor's visits, medication, two instances of hospitalization, and loss of work time by parents who stayed home from jobs to care for their children. On that basis, the 57,345 cases of 1977 billed the country for $17 million.

The success with measles has one limitation: The immunization program has only eliminated the disease as a domestic threat. Infections continue to pop up as visitors from abroad, bearing the virus, enter the U.S. and then infect kids who have not been immunized. For this reason, the CDC will remain in the measles game.

For years, the CDC joined with an international group on the prevention of smallpox. About 200 years ago, Thomas Jefferson, acting as a do-it-yourself physician, inoculated himself, his family, and all of the residents of the estate of Monticello against the disease. At the time, he wrote to Edward Jenner, discoverer of the technique, "Thanks to your work, future generations will know of smallpox only through history."

That great moment finally arrived in 1980 when there was not a single case of that terrible affliction in the entire world. One of the major contributors to the eradication program was Dr. William Foege, who became director of the CDC in 1977. He had devoted fifteen years of his life to the defeat of smallpox. The virus itself still lives, but it is confined to a special lab constructed by the CDC for further research.

In the field of preventive medicine, one of the most fertile territories is that of prenatal and infant care. Dr. Nancy J. Binkin, a Californian, practiced pediatrics and taught at Oakland Children's Hospital and served with medical units in India, Nepal, Kenya, Burma, Thailand, Indonesia, and Sri Lanka before enrolling in the EIS. "I was always interested in public health. I wanted to make more of a contribution than just taking care of kids with running noses. I had a nagging feeling that there must be more to health than that. Primary care [treatment of a patient at the point he or she enters the health-care system] is certainly not the way to go in international health."

As an EIS officer, she spent her first month of duty in an intensive course in Atlanta, learning about the resources available to the organization and studying the principles and methods of field epidemiology. She also took an intensive course in biostatistics, the critical tabulation of facts that provides a portrait of an epidemic.

Almost immediately after completing her training, Binkin was assigned to the Family Planning Unit and was dispatched to Mali, where the government had invited a CDC investigator to assess the effects of illegal abortions. French law still prevailed in Mali, and it proscribed abortion. "The government," says Binkin, "was concerned over the many women hospitalized because of abortions. Among other things these abortions were eating up the country's health budget. I started a study to determine the extent of the abortions and the effects of various methods. Some women took overdoses of antimalarial drugs, which can be very dangerous. Others inserted tree twigs into the vagina, and some women used permanganate to kill the fetus."

But even as Nancy Binkin began to collect the information, a more acute health problem intruded. In the northwest hump of Africa an epidemic of meningococcus flamed up. The ravages of this invisible fire were plain. In Mali's capital, Bamako, 650 cases were reported in a little more than three months, and for the country the figure was 4,000.

As one of the very few trained epidemiologists in Africa at the time, Dr. Binkin was asked by the U.S. Agency for International Development to put her skills to work. She faced a formidable task, not the least of which was the delicate working relationship with the government. "Malians are very proud," says Dr. Binkin. "They are capable people who can do most things themselves. They tend to resent outsiders, and I was never formally invited by the government to work on the meningococcal epidemic."

Binkin and local colleagues were able to institute sanitation measures and gain control over the epidemic. She returned to the U.S., where abortion was legal but where prenatal problems are still very much a factor in the level of national health.

In 1980, at the Sears Corporate Center in Dallas, executives became concerned after the company physician reported a spike in the number of spontaneous abortions among women employees. "Ordinarily," says Binkin, "there are about fifteen of these or neonatal deaths per hundred normal pregnancies. But among the Sears employees the incidence was pegged at eight women in the total of twenty who were pregnant. The Sears management and the physician invited our assistance.

"This is a very difficult kind of investigation," remarks Binkin. "Apart from work there was no common exposure to anything." There has been some talk that video display terminals—VDTs—can have a deleterious effect upon health. "Unfortunately," says Binkin, "twenty women is too small a number for a really scientific survey of this sort of thing. We interviewed the women who lost children, those who had healthy babies. There was no evidence anywhere else to tie VDTs to effects upon health, including spontaneous abortion. Like Love Canal, this sort of thing is very frightening to people but you cannot go on the anecdotal material or ignore the epidemiological statistics."

Subsequently, the spontaneous-abortion rate among pregnant Sears workers in Dallas returned to the statistical norm. Concludes Binkin, "It was necessary to look into the matter; you must rule out possibilities when there is a group with a deviant outcome."

Keeping score is an undramatic but vital element of the CDC's work. When the Atlanta experts, for example, fed into their computers the statistics on deaths connected with reproduction, they learned that the total number of women who died in pregnancy or in efforts to avert pregnancy or childbirth has fallen sharply in recent years. At the same time, deaths caused by contraception (from side effects of the pill and other methods) or sterilization have begun to occur at nearly the same rate as they do in pregnancy itself. The conclusion is that health problems associated with birth control should be studied not because such items as the birth-control pill are more dangerous, but because they are being used by so many more women.

The analysis of the statistics reveals that the fatal effects associated with oral contraceptives are concentrated in women who smoke and those 35 or older. If this segment renounced oral contraception, this method of birth control might be viewed more favorably. Perhaps as startling are findings that the pill has some unexpected good secondary effects, lowering the incidence of certain cancers, reducing iron-deficiency anemias, controlling pelvic inflammations, and even limiting rheumatoid arthritis. The pill may be good for more than prevention of pregnancy.

It would be difficult to find any institution in the U.S. apart from the CDC in a position to gather and analyze such figures. And in these numbers often lie significant information for the betterment of health.

Working with Nancy Binkin on abortion surveillance was Dr. Sally Faith Dorfman. "We're hampered by a lack of data from the states upon which we must depend," says Dorfman. "We're concerned, for example, with ectopic pregnancy, the development of a fetus outside the normal area of the uterus. It can be lethal. The figures indicate 18,000 ectopic pregnancies in 1970 and 42,000 in 1978—the increase more probably due to better reporting than to a sudden surge in the number of defective conceptions. However, with pelvic infections increasing, ectopic pregnancies that scar tissue could subsequently cause more eggs to hang up in a fallopian tube." This is a common pattern for ectopic pregnancies and is life-threatening.

"We need much better statistics," insists Dorfman. "There is a belief that full-term pregnancy is riskless, but the chance of maternal death is not zero—certainly it is not zero after the death of the child before term. At the earliest stages (before three months), abortion is statistically safer than delivery."

Like Binkin, Dorfman investigated a cluster of AROs (adverse reproduction outcomes) in Maryland. The women all worked for a company that raised animals used in lab experiments. When four or five women spontaneously aborted during a relatively short period of time, there was concern over some harmful element in the environment. "Because it was a biological and a scientific environment, the personnel collected data that ordinarily would not be available. The animals were kept free of any environmental contamination or disease. The place was antiseptically clean."

The national average for spontaneous abortion runs between 15 and 20 percent of all pregnancies," points out Dorfman, and it may go from 10 percent one year to 25 percent the next. "We couldn't isolate any cause in Maryland; my feeling is it was just another random occurrence, but it is difficult to rule out possible exposure to some dangerous agent. It may be that a fetus is vulnerable first, but in twenty years, the male employees may develop cancer."

Dorfman was an undergraduate economics major whose interest ran to the social issues of health care, which she describes as "a poorly distributed resource." Doing research on the subject, Dorfman sought out Dr. Leona Baumgartner, a well-known public health expert and then a visiting professor at Harvard. "Baumgartner loved to talk to students, and when I saw her she said, 'If you're serious about health resources, you have got to get your union card. Go to medical school.' " As if that were not enough to tilt Dorfman in the direction of medicine, she was introduced to the man Baumgartner was about to marry, the remarkable Alexander Langmuir, founder of the EIS and then a teacher at Harvard. Langmuir, the dedicated epidemiologist, was also a man of romance; perhaps that quality inspired his protégés as much as his devotion to epidemiology. When Baumgartner had gone off on a trip to Africa, Langmuir had wooed her by having a single red rose waiting for her at every hotel in which she stayed.

"Leona became my professional mother. I checked with her on where to apply, and at one point while we were having dinner, it was Alex who said, 'We should send Sally Faith to the CDC.' "

But it was while Dorfman was in her residency at Beth Israel in Boston that she renewed her acquaintance with another woman doctor, Kay Kreiss, who convinced her finally to apply to the Family Planning Unit at the CDC. "There are certain aspects of the CDC that strike me as like joining the Foreign Legion. It's a good place for people who are at a turning point in their careers and don't know which way to go. For me, it confirmed my interests in the women's health issues and in environmental disease. I've put in four years doing ob gyn, but I don't want to be a full-time private practitioner. I'm looking for jobs that will allow me to work on women's health and the environment at schools of medicine, in international family planning groups. But my CDC experience was wonderful. It's not an oppressive bureaucracy; the people are bright, concerned; nothing gets out unless it's good science. Still, the last year was disappointing—the budget cuts limited travel and investigations; I sense some depression and insecurity in people."

Birth defects also fall under the heading of preventive medicine. Good prenatal care, a proper diet, avoidance of cigarettes, alcohol, and other recreational drugs, and corrective therapy in the face of certain symptoms can reduce the number of youngsters born with physiological problems. Since 1967, the CDC has operated a surveillance program in metropolitan Atlanta looking at newborns, pediatric admissions, spontaneous abortions, and birth defects. Among those involved is Dr. José Cordero, a former EIS officer now on the staff of the Birth Defects Branch of the Chronic Diseases Division.

"It would be extremely useful," says Cordero, "to have a long-term, national study to find factors that might cause birth defects, but it is reasonable to believe that the trends for defects in the five counties around Atlanta reflect the nation. This is an opportunity to see if environmental conditions or drug exposure causes a rise in specific birth defects. We have a system for interviewing the parents and the physicians, getting family history, illnesses, occupations, and the like. One thing that concerns us is that two kinds of cardiovascular birth defects—ventricular septal defect [a hole in the wall of a chamber of the heart] and patent ductus [failure of a fetal channel to close properly after birth]—have doubled over the last ten years. We're also concerned about gathering sufficient data on the effects of prescribed drugs and medicines during pregnancy. What happens to a baby if the mother receives an antibiotic during pregnancy? What about the effect of medicines given to ease morning sickness? You need a lot of cases before you can arrive at any kind of conclusions. We don't have enough personnel to handle a national study. We don't really have enough people for the Atlanta area."

As a father himself, Cordero admits that the possibility of birth defects close to home does cross his mind. Indeed, not long ago, Cordero sat in his living room idly watching his 4-year-old son play with an old stethoscope. "I know what my heart sounds like," announced José Junior. "Lubsh, lubsh."

" 'Come on, José, that's not right,' I said," recalls Cordero.

" 'You're making it up.' But then I took a stethoscope and listened. Sure enough, he was right. My own child had a heart murmur, an innocent one, so small it is no problem, and it was never picked up before even though he's always had the best of medical care. A birth defect is one of the risks of having a child, but you have to take your choice. You can't worry about them. But having a birth defect in my son may help me better understand the effects of the condition upon a family. In José's case, it means such things as having penicillin whenever he goes to the dentist." (While the source of the murmur is unknown, children with cardiovascular defects are more susceptible to dangerous infections.)

Cordero himself had been at the core of a major case involving the health of infants. It began with Dr. Shane Roy III, a specialist in childhood kidney diseases, admitting Peter, a 4-month-old child showing signs of Bartter's disease, an ailment previously found only in adults. The boy's parents had become alarmed when they noticed that their son was not only failing to gain weight but actually was losing a few ounces. A fitful, constipated, and unhappy Peter had visited the family pediatrician several times, but the doctor could not see any reason for the child's lack of appetite and inability to thrive on a diet using a well-established formula food. When Peter's urine began to show traces of blood, the pediatrician recommended that the infant be examined by Dr. Roy at Le Bonheur Hospital.

A laboratory workup under Dr. Roy's supervision uncovered a deficiency of chloride, a vital substance for the health of infants and indeed all humans. The absence of chloride leads to excess acidity in the blood and is known as metabolic alkalosis. The condition is a rare one, occasionally brought on through excessive sweating or prolonged vomiting, and there are nephrologists who never see it during their entire medical career. Over a span of twelve years, Dr. Roy had treated perhaps eight cases.

Dr. Roy prescribed a dietary supplement of potassium chloride to compensate for Peter's deficiency. Within a week, however, a second infant with the same metabolic alkalosis was presented to Dr. Roy, and then a third victim appeared. Like the others he was a child less than 10 months old. The interviews with the parents revealed one common feature:

All three babies ate the same commercially prepared, soy-based formula, Neo-Mull-Soy, manufactured by the Syntex Corporation.

In light of the obvious connection, Dr. Roy immediately notified the Memphis–Shelby County Health Department of both his experience and his suspicions about Neo-Mull-Soy. The health department contacted the CDC on a Friday morning, alerting it to the possibility of an epidemic centering on what was a widely distributed infant food. It was decided that the appropriate section for action was the Birth Defects Branch of the Chronic Diseases Division, and Cordero, then an EIS officer, led the investigation.

Although the preliminary evidence from Dr. Roy tended to indict Neo-Mull-Soy, Cordero's most pressing task was to determine whether cases of metabolic alkalosis among infants existed outside the sale of the baby formula in the Memphis area. Neo-Mull-Soy accounted for about 10 to 12 percent of the soy-based formula market for the country, thousands of infants. The implications of Dr. Cordero's findings would extend well beyond local considerations of health. Should more than a small batch of the stuff sold in one community be found defective—if all of the formula being manufactured and distributed was contaminated or lacked a vital ingredient—the threat to health would be greatly magnified. Also the liability for Syntex could be enormous.

Cordero first heard from Roy on July 26, 1979. Over the next three days, the CDC called a number of pediatric nephrologists and discovered that there were indeed cases of metabolic alkalosis in infants showing up around the country. The common factor was either Neo-Mull-Soy or Cho-Free, another soy-based formula marketed by Syntex. Both substances were prescribed for children who cannot tolerate normal milk products.

The Food and Drug Administration was notified; tests were made of Neo-Mull-Soy and Cho-Free. Both were found to have far less chloride in them than had been recommended in standards of nutrition set by the American Academy of Pediatrics. On the basis of the evidence presented by Cordero, the findings of consulting nephrologists, and its own examination of the formula products, Syntex recalled all Neo-Mull-Soy and Cho-Free on August 1, less than one week after the

CDC had been notified. Syntex explained that a restructuring of its manufacturing process had led to a reduction in the amount of chloride added to the formula.

It was quick work, but more than 130 cases of children suffering from metabolic alkalosis were diagnosed. Whether or not they will suffer permanent damage may not be known until they mature. The recall was not as quick as might have been hoped; there were some 3 million cans of the formula in 57,000 retail establishments. It took months before all were retrieved. Furthermore, the notification process to physicians was spotty; there were parents who, having heard about Neo-Mull-Soy's deficiencies from newspapers, had to insist to hospitals they perform the necessary blood gas inspection to diagnose their sick kids. And even after the formula had been found insufficient, there were pediatricians who continued to insist Neo-Mull-Soy was okay, that the parents were just overly concerned about their child's health. However, when ABC's *20/20* program told the story, the CDC received thousands of telephone calls from worried parents (in marked contrast to the limited number of calls from women worrying about toxic shock syndrome).

Perhaps the most significant result of Cordero's work was the passage of new laws that govern the requirements for infant formula and the quality controls that a company must exercise in order to conform to the rules of the FDA.

The problem with Neo-Mull-Soy stemmed from an error in the recipe for the baby formula. In the clusters of spontaneous abortions investigated by Nancy Binkin and Sally Dorfman the fear was that something in the environment might have terminated the pregnancies. Such cases have inevitably expanded the CDC's charter from its initial preoccupation with communicable diseases to questions about the effects of the environment upon human health.

Dr. Henry Falk, chief of the Chronic Diseases Division's Special Studies Branch, is one of the leaders in studying and investigating the influences upon health of both the natural and man-made environment. Falk is another recruit via the Vietnam War. In his own words, he "blundered into the CDC in 1972." At the time he knew only that he did not wish to be seized by the military draft, and in the course of visiting a friend who sought a public health job, he discovered the CDC.

Much of his work has centered on the hazards of the work site. For example, he investigated a cluster of four cases of angiosarcoma of the liver among workers at a plant manufacturing vinyl chloride. "B.F. Goodrich notified us of the problem," explained Falk. "The job called for workers to clean out these huge pressure cookers. There were no precautions taken; the men were lowered in buckets to chip away at the residues. You could see almost imperceptible changes in the livers over period of time; some men had five biopsies on their livers. Like many of the situations involving toxic chemicals, there are a lot of factors involved. Some people seem to metabolize substances differently; some people excrete the toxins faster than others. There are a lot of enzymes in the body that normally detoxify chemicals, but sometimes they don't do the job and the stuff becomes a carcinogen.

"We weren't notified until after the third case of angiosarcoma was diagnosed; whether it would have made any difference if we had been called earlier, I can't say. Certainly the company doctor was extremely cooperative once we began our investigation. In Europe, where the same problem occurred, there had been a suspicion that the chemical companies were more aware of problems than they let on."

Based on the CDC investigation led by Falk, the practices for cleaning the tanks were changed. Workers no longer were lowered into the vats to chip away the residues.

Falk worked on another vinyl-chloride problem when meat wrappers in a supermarket began to develop asthma. At some costs to the industry, the meat-wrapping technique was changed, reducing the opportunities for employees to inhale fumes hazardous to their health.

José Cordero actually was working in Falk's unit when he led the investigation that resulted in the recall of Neo-Mull-Soy. Another EIS officer under Falk's command, Dr. Kay Kreiss, did the fieldwork when the mayor of a small Alabama town, Triana, asked for assistance because the local citizens showed elevated levels of DDT in their blood, the result of toxic-waste dumping in the local river, which had put the chemical in the food chain.

Sometimes natural cataclysms become the target for an investigation by Falk's people in the Chronic Diseases Division. Dr. Edwin Kilbourne was an EIS officer during the 1980 heat wave in the central part of the United States when about 1,200 deaths were attributed to the prolonged spell of hot weather; seventeen days passed with the thermometer going over 102°. The phenomenon provided epidemiologists with an opportunity to study the effects of heat. Not surprisingly, poor people suffered more. The upper floors of tenements, which had neither air conditioning nor shade trees, cooked human cells at a frightening rate. Kilbourne learned that people over 65 years of age are more than twelve times as much at risk as those younger. Blacks were felled from heat stroke more than whites, but that fact may have less to do with racial physiology than economics.

The data from that study provided a possible base line for future action. It indicated at what floor level in a building residents should be evacuated in the event of severe heat. It raised questions on where temperatures should be measured. Typically, measuring is done at airports, but perhaps attention should be directed to areas and buildings where the heat is retained, making for exposure at higher levels over more extended periods of time. There's no question that cities are far riskier than suburbs. In St. Louis, the death rate was triple that of the rest of the state.

Thus, one of the CDC's future missions may lie in input for urban planning, for matters of public construction and transportation. However, questions about environmental impact upon health are so new, and as yet so ill defined, that a number of different CDC units are engaged in hunting for information. Consider the case of Globe, Arizona, and the homes built upon land impregnated with asbestos wastes.

Asbestos fibers were among the earliest substances clearly shown to be hazardous to lungs. The most common form of the mineral, chrysotile asbestos, is considered both fibrogenic and carcinogenic. The former indicates that it produces asbestosis, in which the alveola—the minute sacs of the lungs—become clogged and fibrous. As a carcinogen, asbestos may cause cancer of the lungs or mesothelioma, a cancerous disease of the lining that protectively envelops the lungs. It is also a process that shows itself relatively slowly, plugging the lung sacs over a long period of time, from fifteen to twenty years before either cancer appears or emphysema, a degenerative, progressively worse condition, slowly suffocates a person.

In October 1979, a state sewer inspector made a routine examination of a development called Mountain View Mobile Home Estates, some 2 miles from Globe, Arizona, a copper-mining center. The development was located in the midst of some asbestos-processing plants. While examining the drainage system, the sewer expert fell into conversation with one of the residents, who idly pointed to a fine gray-white substance heaped in mounds scattered around the development. The homeowner remarked that the stuff was asbestos tailings. Wasn't that supposed to be dangerous?

Aware of the reputation of asbestos, the sewer inspector promptly carried the news back to his superiors. Dr. Alex Kelter, at the time employed by the Arizona State Department of Health Services and later to become an EIS officer who worked with Jim Curran on the case of the gay men's disease (see Chapter 4), was assigned to look at the site.

"The subdivision had had repeated problems with its sewage-disposal system," says Kelter. "The inspector had reported, 'There were gobs of material hanging from the roofs, blowing through the yards. Kids had gotten inside one of the buildings, played with the equipment, spread asbestos fibers outside. When we arrived, the mill operators gave us a tour; they were sort of proud of the piles of tailings, the amount of production. We saw big uncovered heaps; there was a sprinkler system around to wet it down, prevent it from blowing about. Some of the people there insisted the sprinklers had just been installed before our visit. Parents told us the kids used to make asbestos snowballs, throw them at one another, stuff them down inside each other's shirts."

Alex Kelter telephoned the CDC's Dr. Clark Heath, director of the Chronic Diseases Division, and described the asbestos exposures at Globe. Dr. Roy Ing, an EIS officer in the Cancer Branch, was dispatched to Arizona for an on-site inspection.

Ing was accompanied to the Mountain View site by Dr. James Lemen, a physician attached to the National Institute for Occupational Safety and Health (NIOSH), a subsidiary of the CDC. NIOSH sent Lemen because the source of the tailings was the mills and there was concern over whether these were continuing to pollute the area as well as questions about the work conditions for those still laboring in the mills.

How Mountain View arrived at its condition is a tale of industry investment and government action and inaction, and of human beings spurred by their particular interests and passions. What occurred at Globe indicated some of the difficulties that the CDC must confront if it moves deeper into environmental health, particularly where economics are involved.

Originally there were three mills on the site, processing chrysolite asbestos from nearby mines. The plants removed the commercially useful longer fibers by blowing crushed ore through a series of filters. The ore residues, called tailings, and which still contained an abundance of shorter and unwanted fibers, usually were dumped in piles beside the mills.

Starting in 1971, L. C. Kopisch, director of the local Pinal-Gila Air Pollution District, had registered objections to the dust emissions from the mills. He skirmished with the mill companies and their lawyers for two years. Just when Kopisch thought he had achieved his goal and secured a court order shutting the plants down, Congressman John B. Conlan, on behalf of the mill operators, appealed to the federal Environmental Protection Agency. An EPA office in San Francisco, 1,000 miles away, issued an approval for the mills to continue operations. The EPA had surveyed the area near Globe only when the plants were not operating. The inspectors never saw any excessive emissions.

Kopisch was outraged and wrote to the EPA regional director: "I wish you would explain in clear language just what in the hell you think you are doing." Kopisch managed to obtain another injunction against the mills unless emission controls were improved. Two of them complied. The third was owned by the Metate Asbestos Corporation. Its operator, Jack Neal, had announced earlier he would not spend "one cent on emission control," and he proved a man of his word. Kopisch refused to issue a permit to Metate, but a year later, after complaints from people, he discovered that the place was still processing ore. The air-pollution official procured the necessary papers to ensure a halt to mill operations.

But a year earlier, Jack Neal and his wife had managed to get the property zoned for residential use and were selling lots in a development, Mountain View Mobile Home Estates, that surrounded the now defunct mill.

By 1979, thirty-eight families with a total population of 118 people had moved into the community. When Roy Ing arrived on the scene, he found in the center of the mobile home sites an abandoned mill with asbestos wastes strewn about it. Inside the shut-down building there were machines thick with asbestos dust.

In forty-four of the fifty building lots, the investigators determined that 5 percent of the soil was asbestos. Four samples registered 50 percent asbestos. The chrysolite fibers showed up in dust drawn from furnace filters and from vacuum-cleaner bags. Airborne asbestos fibers in concentrations as high as 4,000 fibers per cubic meter were detected in both indoor and outdoor air. Much higher levels of concentrations were registered in sampling devices used by the residents.

The Occupational Safety and Health Administration (OSHA) had set a limit of 2 million fibers per cubic meter as an eight-hour, time-weighted average, although NIOSH and the CDC recommended that it be lowered, substantially, to 100,000 fibers per cubic meter. However, the occupational standard was designed for someone on a job in a mill or mine, working with asbestos. It was never intended to be an outer limit for anyone exposed twenty-four hours a day with no asbestos-free air to inspire. Certainy it was never designed as the allowable level for kids playing on a pile of asbestos tailings. Ing considered the asbestos-fiber content of the air intolerably high.

When the mill site was originally prepared as a housing development, the tailings had been used as fill, and 6 inches of topsoil was trucked in and spread to cover the contaminated layers beneath. But every subsequent trench made for drainage, every shrub or tree that required a hole 6 inches or deeper, dug up the asbestos remnants. Wind and natural erosion combined to carry away some of the covering topsoil, and of course there were the heaps of discarded materials around the mill site.

As an immediate therapy for the wounded development,

William Foege, director of the CDC, urged the state to evacuate those living at Mountain View Homes and to decontaminate the subdivision. Subsequently, the governor of Arizona authorized temporary housing for the people at Mountain View while their properties were decontaminated. The families were told to launder all of their garments and wipe all belongings with wet cloths before taking off for their temporary digs.

The initial reports from the Arizona Division of Occupational Safety and Health and from NIOSH moved Governor Bruce Babbit to promise residents, "If that building [the mill] is standing in six months, I will mobilize the National Guard to tear it down, board by board and brick by brick."

The mill building was demolished, its pieces buried. Another 6 inches of topsoil covered open ground, which was seeded. But heavy rains during the spring washed away some of the new earth, exposing anew the contaminated soil.

For his part, Jack Neal saw no reason for the fuss. "We still don't feel it's a health hazard. Our children grew up with it." The residents found themselves in a bind. The publicity had destroyed any chances of selling out and moving to a healthier area. Yet at this point they could not demonstrate any illnesses that could be clearly traced to asbestos. The Mountain View development had been inhabited for only eight years, which might be too short a period for lungs to show damage from the asbestos. Most of the residents had lived there for a considerably shorter time.

Jan Ianello has resided there for six years and was among those visited by Roy Ing. "All we noticed was that we seem to have a lot of sinus and respiratory conditions, irritations. From the time they discovered the problem we've had physicals from the state and even sputum tests [to determine whether any dust has reached the lungs]. Dr. Ing was very upset and concerned. He wanted us out of here immediately. The kids complained often about itchy eyes.

"But we weren't aware of all of the stuff. We didn't notice it because it was behind a large building. All they had out front was in bags. I heard they were supposed to keep sprinkling it, wet it down, but it gets so dry around here that the water doesn't do much to keep the fibers from blowing around. Three families got up and left; one man had to move because his doctor said he had cancer of the lungs. Dr. Ing told us our homes were contaminated. We saw a program on TV and we learned that the fibers can penetrate the skin; you don't have to ingest it. We know it is dangerous but we just sit; nobody wants to buy our house."

Recalls Alex Kelter, "We found people with illnesses, nothing directly attributed to asbestos, except a heck of a lot of anxiety. Several dozen of them smoked cigarettes; that, of course, is a big multiplier of lung problems when coupled with exposure of asbestos. There was a lot of anger, frustration, but there was no quick solution. The affair raises the question of how much responsibility a government has to certify that a piece of land is habitable; unless you know about prior usage, the legal and illegal dump of toxic substances, you're going to be shooting in the dark."

This experience was one of several Kelter had with the CDC, and it led him to apply to the EIS. "I was interested in environmental hazards, and I thought in the CDC I'd get an opportunity to concentrate in that field. The EIS was rewarding in that I could work in epidemiology without a lot of administrative stuff—budgets, supervisors, reports. Still, it wasn't what I expected. So much was in service to states, and the ability to deal with a problem depends on a hit-and-miss system where we find out about something by happenstance and then must wangle an invitation to come in." When his career in the EIS ended, Kelter accepted a post in the Chronic Diseases Division of the CDC.

Roy Ing's reaction to Globe was intense. "I was appalled at what I saw," says Ing. "This stuff was everywhere. My initial impression was that no one should continue to live there. It wasn't just the exposure when somebody went outside; the homes were all contaminated by dust carried in on clothes and shoes or it blew in through open windows and doors."

At this point, all Ing and his colleagues can do is monitor the health of those who remain at Mountain View Estates. But perhaps because of his Chinese background, the San Francisco–born physician has always been oriented toward preventive medicine, and that makes a situation like Globe even more frustrating.

Both as an EIS officer and in other investigations, however, Ing has been able to work on problems that do not require

years of waiting before coming up with findings. For instance, he was assigned to look into the process by which
materials were manufactured for log-cabin homes in Lexington, Kentucky. "The technique," explains Ing, "was to dip the
logs in vats of pentachlorophenol. It's the same stuff used on
utility poles, except that there it was done under pressure. For
the logs in homes, they only wanted penetration of about a
quarter of an inch, enough to control sap stain and prevent
funguses and insects like wood borers or even bumble bees."

In 1979, however, the Department of Agriculture reported
that cattle which chewed on wooden posts impregnated with
the chemical died. Although some log-cabin makers immediately switched to another substance, others continued to use
pentachlorophenol. Ing's investigation was concerned with
the possible effects upon factory hands, and again he was
working with representatives of NIOSH.

"While we were looking at the factory in Kentucky," says
Ing, "we received a telephone call from someone living in
Lexington. He said he'd heard of our research and since he
lived in one of the log homes he wondered whether there was
any danger to his family and himself." Tests on residents of
homes constructed from logs with pentachlorophenol did
indicate concentrations of toxic chemicals in their blood-
streams. As a consequence of Ing's studies, the procedures
for manufacturing were changed and a long-term surveillance
project to monitor people living in pentachlorophenol-tainted
environments established. "The problem," notes Ing, "is we
may not know for many years whether there is a real hazard."

Ing was among those dispatched to the scene of a natural
but abrupt change in environment, the eruption of Mt. St.
Helens. "We worked with federal and state agencies on a
number of matters. We studied those who died and who survived in the vicinity of the mountain. We looked at the ash
fall from the eruption, plotting where it went. We checked
the emergency-room visits, the respiration problems of patients, hospital admissions, and death rates in the months after
the eruption." Along with the investigation by Ing, NIOSH
focused upon loggers who had the task of returning to the
surrounding slopes to salvage lumber. The scientists were
concerned about the possible long-term effects of working in
an environment so heavily charged with ash, which causes

fibrosis or scarring of the lungs. The cutting of timber, the machines, even the loggers' boots would stir up clouds of ash and small particles that are a known cause of fibrosis. One result of the NIOSH inspection was a requirement for the loggers to wear masks.

Ing and company also tried to determine what had actually killed the people trapped by the eruption. A number of deaths proved to be not from the fierce heat and fire of the blast but from the inhalation of ash—asphyxia. Some people survived although closer to the blast than a number who died. The people who lived saved themselves by protecting their airways, jumping into streams to avoid burns and shielding their airways by pulling a wet T-shirt over their heads.

The experts also discovered signs of legionella after the eruption. Such violent upheavals of the earth may be responsible for churning up bacteria, raising the risk of epidemic disease.

In 1982, the person most heavily charged with guiding the CDC was tall—basketball-height at least—and unflappable Dr. William Foege. He assumed command of the CDC after Dr. David Sencer lost his position in 1977 because then HEW Secretary Joseph Califano thought the agency was becalmed, perhaps doomed to stagnation because of the blunders with the ill-fated swine flu program. (Most people at the CDC during Sencer's regime regarded him as a dynamic force, albeit occasionally insensitive to the feelings of associates and other government officials.)

But when Bill Foege, himself a former EIS officer, looks at the public health of America he sees other routes than simple inoculations and cleaning up the environment. "When my father was born, diphtheria was the third leading cause of death among children. Last year only one such death occurred. That's an indication of how health concerns must change. The CDC's objectives are to reduce unnecessary morbidity [sickness] and premature mortality and to improve the quality of life, hardly a program that anyone could quarrel with." But toward that goal a HEW task force that included Foege arranged for letters to be mailed to more than 1,000 people—movers, shakers, and public health experts—for their notions of the ways to approach these objectives. Then eighteen top experts on health, unconnected with the government, met to look at sickness, death, and the arts of prevention. "We asked them to tell us the twelve most important things to do toward prevention," recalls Foege. "They wouldn't 'prioritize' the twelve but gave us an alphabetical list." Foege ticks off some of the points of departure if major advances in health are to be achieved.

"Smoking and alcohol are associated with the two biggest cancers—lung and cervical. These fall within the power of prevention, intervention. Smoking and alcohol are also critical in terms of cardiovascular health. About 1,000 people die prematurely each day from cigarettes. We added three items to the dozen the panel gave us—unwanted pregnancy, environmental health, and violence. [Other topics were control of high blood pressure, pregnancy, immunization, sexually transmitted diseases, toxic-agent control, accident prevention and injury control, fluoridation and dental health, surveillance and control of infectious diseases, nutrition, physical fitness, and exercise.] It is possible to look upon homicides and accidents as preventable deaths. Violence is preventable, but not so long as it is seen only as something for law enforcement only to deal with. If epidemiologists were to work full-time on the problem of violence as a public health problem, a self-inflicted disease in many instances, there might be some significant achievements.

"Alcohol is involved in a third of all accidental deaths; other countries have programs that have reduced the alcohol-related deaths substantially. Getting support for that kind of a program by the CDC and the government is much different from one for polio. With alcohol there are vested interests. There are many things in homes and work places also. Building codes could mandate smoke detectors to protect against burns. The number of people scalded by hot water could be greatly reduced if there were thermostats that did not allow water above 105°." Changing these circumstances to prevent the "diseases" they can produce is quite different from inoculating kids against diphtheria.

"In medical school I realized that resources never meet needs, and by that principle, prevention is the most efficient route to better health," says Foege. "Most medical resources are in the Western World, while the majority of needs lie in the Third World. Prevention in the Third World is even more important."

Even while ruminating on this grand vision of health concerns, Foege hastens to add, "We still cannot reduce our input into anthrax, just because it's so rare a disease. No one else is qualified to do what we've been doing."

The 1983 budget for the CDC is set at $217 million, up $5 million from the previous year but substantially below the $300 million of peak years. Some of this reduction is misleading, since what was taken out of the appropriation was largely in the area of the block grants to the states, formerly administered by the CDC for preventive programs. Whether the states will, under the new federalism, be able to make up for the decline in money for programs in fluoridation, lead-poisoning control, and other operations remains questionable. Paul Blake, who hunted down the source of Louisiana's cholera outbreaks (see Chapter 3), talks about the magnificent work done by local public health personnel, whose operations may be seriously curtailed because of the loss of appropriations.

At one point it appeared that the CDC was going to be forced to trim its staff by 700 people, which would have meant a severe reduction in epidemiological studies and small numbers of EIS officers. However, funds to cover this type of work were restored. Less fortunate has been NIOSH. This unit of the CDC has always dealt heavily in grants to local authorities charged with keeping the work place healthy. Not only has the NIOSH portion of the money been drastically cut, but also the prevailing attitude in the national administration is for less interference in the workings of business and industry. As a consequence, NIOSH is barely a factor and the morale on the staff is low.

For all of its successes, the future of the CDC is by no means assured. Bruce Dan argues that were it not for cost-consciousness, the CDC labs would have pursued the mechanism of toxic shock and come up with a definitive answer on the role of super-absorbent tampons. Others at the CDC rebut Dan and claim there was already ongoing research in state institutions. The CDC's expertise was thus unnecessary. But again, the state hospitals and universities are not as well equipped as the CDC and they too have fiscal troubles.

The on-again, off-again reductions in force and operations have confused and frustrated CDC people. Donald Francis, the hepatitis expert, growls, "If they'd just leave us alone, we'd be better off."

Under the new federalism it would seem logical to leave the work of the CDC to local governments, universities, even private foundations. That was indeed the way before the CDC. The final isolation of yellow fever virus in Africa came from a team working on a Rockefeller Foundation grant in 1927. Yet, disease rarely halts at the city, county, or state borders; only someone with a mandate for the entire country can effectively pursue the epidemiology to its logical end. Legionnaires' disease is a case in point.

There is, of course, another federal organization that has long been interested in investigations of disease—the military. The involvement there began as crude biological warfare, U.S. Army units giving smallpox-ridden blankets to Indians and putting the corpses of diseased cattle into Confederate wells. There was a shift when the U.S. temporarily occupied Cuba after the Spanish-American War and valiant efforts were made to find the cause of yellow fever. Several human guinea pigs in the military were casualties. The information, however, proved vital not only for Cuba, but also for the subsequent building of the Panama Canal. The French had been defeated not by geography but by yellow fever.

The military went back into the disease business during World War II. Malaria was a major problem for troops in the South Pacific, venereal disease on the home front and in occupied territories.

The military did not quit the field after V-J Day, however, although the Center for Communicable Diseases had been established to deal with malaria and other threats to troops. The difference now was that the military was less interested in protecting its fighting forces than in figuring whether diseases could serve as weapons. At Fort Detrick, Maryland, a biological-warfare unit was established. It's been at work ever since, studying things like anthrax, botulism, and bubonic plague as potential thunderbolts.

The work at Fort Detrick has some affinity with certain aspects of CDC studies; the effectiveness of a biological weapon depends upon how swiftly it can be spread, how deadly it will be, how quickly it will render victims helpless, and what kinds of countermeasures the enemy can take. The same questions must also be answered by specialists assigned to worry about what may happen to U.S. forces if a foe resorts to viruses, bacteria, or toxins.

There has been some movement of people between the CDC and Fort Detrick—Joe McDade, who first saw legionella, for example, and Karl Johnson, the expert on hemorrhagic diseases. However, there are health experts who do fear that the CDC might come uncomfortably close to the work at Fort Detrick, compromising the reputation of the CDC and even destroying its welcome abroad as a worldwide resource.

No one accuses the CDC of collusion in germ warfare. But there is an uneasy feeling, much the same as that in law-enforcement circles when a prosecutor leaves office, taking with him his knowledge of policies and intelligence and possibly putting them at the service of those with interests opposed to those of law enforcement.

When Atlanta and indeed the entire country grew fearful over the deaths of a number of young Atlantans, the CDC offered its epidemiological expertise toward a solution. (Criminal and medical detection met at a logical intersection.) The CDC's proposal quickly became an element in a sad farce as social critic Dick Gregory propounded the theory that the children were the victims of a CDC experiment, an attempt to develop immunity against cancer for aging white people by means of the tissue from the penises of the dead black children.

For weeks the CDC fended off telephone calls from inquiring reporters. The affair was climaxed by a Philadelphia radio show on which the CDC's official spokesman, Don Berreth, wound up debating with Gregory. Ultimately, Berreth invited Gregory to come to Atlanta with his proof, and Gregory duly showed up with attorney Mark Lane, who had been uncharacteristically invisible since he had pronounced the Rev. Jim Jones (just before the Guyana mass suicide) a heroic leader. Gregory's evidence amounted to a pastiche of newspaper clippings on medical experiments conducted by the military with hallucinogens and other agents. There was absolutely nothing to connect the CDC with the murders.

In a way, the affair suggests how treacherous the future for the CDC may be. While it is unlikely that it will have to contend often with such ridiculous charges as Gregory's, major advances in the directions suggested by Foege may lead it away from the neat, dramatic successes against infections and into thickets of big-city politics, racisms, manners and mores, and vested economic interests. Putting out the invisible fires of infection is tough enough; doing so while others may surreptitiously or openly be feeding gasoline to the blaze could be something that might even endanger the firefighters themselves.

BIBLIOGRAPHY

Archer, Jules, *Epidemic*. Harcourt Brace, 1977.

Beveridge, I. B., *Influenza, The Last Great Plague*. Prodist, 1977.

Cahill, Kevin M. (editor), *The AIDS Epidemic*. St. Martin's Press, 1983.

Collier, Richard, *The Plague of the Spanish Lady*. Atheneum, 1974.

Fuller, John G., *Fever, The Hunt for a New Killer Virus*. Reader's Digest Books, 1974.

Gottfried, Robert, *The Black Death*. Free Press, Collier Macmillan, 1982.

Imperato, Pascal James, *Medical Detective*. R. Marek, 1979.

Kassler, Jeanne, *Gay Men's Health*. Harper & Row, 1983.

Kruif, Paul de, *Microbe Hunters*. Harcourt Brace Jovanovich, 1926.

McNeill, William Hardy, *Plagues and Peoples*. Anchor Press, 1976.

Rosenberg, Howard, *Atomic Soldiers*. Beacon Press, 1980.

Roueché, Berton, *Eleven Blue Men*. Little, Brown & Co., 1953.

———*The Incurable Wound*. Little, Brown & Co., 1957.

———*The Orange Man*. Little, Brown & Co., 1971.

———*The Medical Detectives*. Times Books, 1980.

Thomas, Gordon, and Morgan-Witts, Max, *Anatomy of an Epidemic*. Doubleday, 1982.

Uhl, Michael, *GI Guinea Pigs*. Playboy Press, 1980.

Whiteside, Thomas, *The Pendulum and the Toxic Cloud*. Yale University Press, 1978.

Zinsser, Hans, *Rats, Lice and History*. Little, Brown & Co., 1935.

Index

217